PRAISE FOR The IBS Guide

"Nicely written; thorough; up to date. Carefully crafted chapters review treatment options demonstrated to improve IBS symptoms, including dietary interventions, alternative therapies, over-the-counter agents, prescription medications and psychological therapies. This book is a must read for those who want to know more about IBS and for those who want better control of their IBS symptoms."

- Brian Lacy, Ph.D., M.D., FACG, Professor of Medicine
Program Director, GI Fellowship, Mayo Clinic, Jacksonville
Author, *"Making Sense of IBS"*

"This is an excellent, informative and comprehensive work. It is a great example that knowledge is power and should be part of every patient's armamentarium against IBS."

- Daniel C. DeMarco, M.D., FACP, FACG, AGAF, FASGE
Professor of Medicine, Texas A&M College of Medicine
Current President, Texas Club of Internists
Former Advisor to the CPT Editorial Panel of the
American Medical Association

"Patients looking for an easy-to-read, practical, and thorough source of the latest information about IBS need go no further than Dr. Kethu's superb book. Written in straightforward English, its 18 chapters present everything that a patient needs to know, from suspected causes to diagnosis and management. Therapy is discussed in detail, including diet, both standard and complementary medications, and psychological approaches. Actionable advice about coping strategies is presented. The reader will better understand the condition, have more realistic expectations about available treatments, and be able to grasp how to live a full life despite their diagnosis. I recommend that every person with IBS reads this book."

- Lawrence R. Schiller, M.D., MACG
Clinical Professor, Department of Medical Education
Texas A&M University School of Medicine, Dallas Campus
Past President, American College of Gastroenterology

The IBS Guide

The IBS Guide

Explore the Mind, Gut, Microbiome and
A Holistic Approach to Conquer IBS

Sripathi Kethu, M.D.

Forestbrook Publishers

The IBS Guide:

Explore the Mind, Gut, Microbiome and A Holistic Approach to Conquer IBS

Disclaimer:

The information in this book is for educational purposes only and should not be considered medical advice or a substitute for professional healthcare. The author and publisher have tried to ensure accuracy, but medical knowledge and research are constantly evolving.

This book is not intended to diagnose, treat, cure, or prevent any disease or condition. Consult your healthcare provider before changing your diet, life-style, or treatment plan. The author and publisher are not responsible for any adverse effects resulting from the information in this book.

Individual experiences with irritable bowel syndrome may vary. Consult a healthcare professional before making any changes to your healthcare plan. The author and publisher disclaim liability for any loss, damage, or injury that may occur due to the use or misuse of the information in this book.

ISBN: 979-8-9883598-0-7 (Print)
ISBN: 979-8-9883598-1-4 (eBook)

Dedication

*My parents, for their unwavering support and
unconditional love that shaped my life*

*My wife, Sireesha, for standing by my side through every
high and low, and for being my rock*

*Samira and Sumana, our wonderful daughters,
who fill our lives with love and joy*

Foreword

Irritable bowel syndrome affects 1 in 10 adult Americans. Chronic IBS symptoms can interfere with social events, disrupt daily life activities at home and work, and greatly reduce the overall quality of life for the millions who struggle with this frustrating disorder. Fortunately, a host of treatment options are now available to improve chronic symptoms of constipation, diarrhea, abdominal pain, and bloating.

In "The IBS Guide", Dr. Kethu, an experienced gastroenterologist, reviews the causes of IBS, explains why symptoms develop, and discusses appropriate diagnostic tests. Carefully crafted chapters review treatment options demonstrated to improve IBS symptoms, including dietary interventions, alternative therapies, over-the-counter agents, prescription medications, and psychological therapies.

This book is a must-read for those who want to know more about IBS and for those who want better control of their IBS symptoms.

Brian E. Lacy, Ph.D., M.D., FACG
Professor of Medicine
Associate Program Director, Scholarly Activities
Program Director, GI Fellowship
Consultant
Mayo Clinic, Jacksonville

A Note from the Author

Did you know that irritable bowel syndrome (IBS) affects 10-20% of the global population, with 25-45 million people in the US alone? While it is true that IBS is not a deadly condition, it can take a significant toll on the physical and emotional health of those suffering from it.

Healthcare costs for IBS are substantial, with direct medical expenses and indirect costs like absenteeism from work and decreased productivity. IBS can also affect social life, mental health, and emotional well-being, causing patients to avoid social events, travel, and eating out. They may feel embarrassed or ashamed of their condition, leading to anxiety and depression. Many struggle in silence believing that there is no solution. As a gastroenterologist with over two decades of experience treating patients with IBS, I have seen firsthand the devastating impact this condition can have on those suffering from it.

Over the course of my career, I have observed how utilizing evidence-based methods, making dietary changes, and one's lifestyle can significantly enhance the quality of life for individuals with IBS. I am grateful for the opportunity to have impacted the lives of thousands of patients through my clinical practice. I created this comprehensive guide with the goal of reaching a larger audience and helping others. It provides valuable insights for those seeking answers.

You may be wondering, "With so many books already available on IBS and a wealth of free information online, why do we need yet another book on this topic?" Well, that is the exact reason why I wrote this book! There is too much information for a lot of us to digest!! (pun intended).

As a healthcare provider, I have noticed that my patients research quite a bit about this condition. Still, they come back to me with more questions than answers because it is sometimes hard to tease out facts from fiction and anecdotes from objective scientific evidence. In the wise words of John Nesbit, an American author and futurist, "We are drowning in information but starved for knowledge." This sentiment inspired me to write this guide on IBS that presents the latest research in a clear and easy-to-understand manner.

This book thoroughly explores the causes of IBS by delving into the gut-brain relationship, visceral hypersensitivity, microbiome, gut motility, family history, stress, and postinfectious IBS. We will also address controversial topics like leaky gut and Candida of the gut, and offer holistic management techniques for IBS, including diets, meal planning, and mind-body methods such as cognitive behavioral therapy, hypnotherapy, yoga, meditation, and exercise.

We will evaluate over the counter and prescription medications, complementary therapies, and digital apps. Additionally, we have included a 28-day meal plan created by a registered dietician. Furthermore, we will address specific challenges, such as IBS in women and bloating, discuss coping strategies and support sources, and offer tips for living a full life while managing IBS at work, during travel, and socially. Lastly, we will consider the future of IBS patients, including new insights into causes, diagnostic methods, and emerging therapies like neurostimulation and digital technologies that will revolutionize IBS care.

IBS is a condition that should not be underestimated. However, with the proper knowledge and tools, those with IBS can regain control of their lives and live without constant symptoms. This book is a valuable resource for individuals with IBS, their loved ones, and healthcare providers. It provides a comprehensive understanding of the science behind the symptoms and offers practical guidance for managing IBS to improve overall health. Patient success stories are included to inspire hope and offer guidance for various clinical scenarios.

This book aims to provide accurate, concise, up-to-date, and practical information to help you effectively manage your IBS. By improving gut health and empowering individuals to live free from debilitating IBS symptoms, we aim to positively impact the lives of many affected by IBS.

Welcome to our journey towards better gut health and overall well-being. I wish you great health and happiness.

Table of Contents

CHAPTER 1

Introduction to Irritable Bowel Syndrome

"Health is not valued till sickness comes." - Thomas Fuller

Definition and overview

Before discussing irritable bowel syndrome (IBS), it is important to understand functional gastrointestinal disorder (FGID), which is now called "disorders of gut-brain interaction" (DGBI). This condition occurs when there is a disturbance in the digestive system, but tests and scans do not show any clear issues. Some common examples of DGBI include IBS, functional dyspepsia, and functional heartburn.

There are multiple factors that can lead to DGBIs, including genetics, gut sensitivity, motility, and stress. Doctors usually diagnose DGBIs based on symptoms and treat them with a combination of dietary adjustments, lifestyle changes, psychotherapy, and medications. IBS is a specific type of digestive disorder that affects the small and large intestines. Common symptoms of IBS include abdominal pain, gas, bloating, and changes to bowel habits such as diarrhea, constipation, or both.

The History of IBS: understanding the evolution of the condition

Although IBS may appear to be a modern ailment, it has been documented throughout history. The ancient civilizations of Egypt, Greece, and Rome recorded symptoms similar to IBS. For instance, the Ebers

Papyrus, an ancient Egyptian medical document from 1500 BCE, describes gastrointestinal issues and irregular bowel movements that resemble IBS symptoms.

Hippocrates, the renowned Greek physician known as the "Father of Medicine," documented symptoms similar to IBS in 400 BCE. He believed in maintaining a balance of the body's four humors - blood, phlegm, yellow bile, and black bile - to ensure that everything, including our digestive system, worked smoothly.

Fast forward to the 2nd century AD, the Roman doctor Galen also mentioned IBS-like symptoms. Over time, people used different names for IBS-like issues, like "mucous colitis," which Sir William Osler came up with in 1892. These early observations have contributed to our understanding of IBS today.

In the early 1900s, IBS went by a bunch of names like "spastic colon," "colitis," and "nervous stomach," but they didn't quite hit the mark. A spastic colon is about colon spasms, which is only part of IBS. Colitis means colon inflammation, which is not the main issue in IBS. A nervous stomach is when stress or anxiety messes with your gut. Sure, stress can trigger IBS, but it is not the only reason.

In the mid-1900s, the term "irritable bowel syndrome" was coined to describe a set of gut symptoms lacking a clear cause. To better diagnose and treat this condition, doctors developed criteria such as the Manning criteria in the 1970s and the Rome criteria in the 1990s.

The history of IBS shows considerable progress in understanding and managing this complicated condition. Initially, doctors believed that it was solely caused by anxiety or stress, but we now understand that IBS is a complex interplay of several factors.

Prevalence of IBS

IBS affects around 10-15% of people in the US. That is over 25-45 million people! It is one of the most common gut problems doctors come across in their practice. IBS cases are growing worldwide, with 10-20% of people affected depending on the country. It is hard to nail down exact numbers because it varies by how each country handles IBS cases and what kind of diagnostic criteria they have used. Here is a snapshot of IBS prevalence rates around the globe:

- Mexico: 15-20%
- Canada: 18%
- United States: 10-15%
- Europe: 10-15% (varies by country, up to 20% in some places)
- Colombia: 6.3-16.3%
- India: 14%
- China: 5-14% (higher in urban areas)
- Japan: 5-15% (higher in women and elderly)
- Brazil: 4.4-15.6%
- Russia: 12.8%
- Saudi Arabia: 12.4%
- Pakistan: 11.6%
- Africa: 6-10% (varies by country, higher in urban areas)

More women get IBS than men, with 1.5 to 3 times higher rates. We are not sure if it is biology or social factors causing this. A large study from 2022 found that 16% of medical staff worldwide have IBS. Things like shift work, lousy sleep, and being a woman made it more likely, so stress and gender do play a role in IBS. Another study in 2023 showed that a whopping 25% of US army veterans have IBS, and it is even higher (39%) among female vets. Risk factors for vets include stress, anxiety, depression, and exposure to gastrointestinal infections. In another study of army veterans, IBS rates jumped from 10% before deployment to 30% after, again showing that infections and stressful situations matter.

Who is at risk for IBS?

IBS can affect anyone, but certain factors may increase the risk of developing the condition. Some of these factors include:

1. **Age:** IBS is more common in people under 50, but it can affect individuals of all ages.
2. **Gender:** Women are more likely to be diagnosed with IBS than men. This may be due, in part, to hormonal differences or a greater willingness for women to seek medical care for their symptoms.
3. **Family history:** If you have a close family member with IBS, your chances of developing the condition may be higher.
4. **Stress and psychological factors:** Stress, anxiety, and depression are common triggers for IBS symptoms. Individuals who have experienced traumatic events or have a history of mental health issues may be more susceptible to developing IBS.

Why is IBS important?

Impact on quality of life: IBS symptoms can be a real pain and mess with your life. They can throw off your daily routine and get in the way of work, school, and hanging out with friends.

Social stigma: IBS can make people feel embarrassed or self-conscious, leading to social isolation and feeling bad about themselves.

This can cause shame, guilt, or embarrassment and might make people keep to themselves or avoid getting help.

Mental health: IBS can also hurt mental health, with higher rates of depression, anxiety, and other problems than those without IBS.

Economic burden: IBS can hit your wallet hard, both for you and the society in general. Healthcare costs for IBS in the US alone are estimated at $1.6 billion per year, covering doctor visits, tests, and medications. Indirect costs like missing work and lost productivity are enormous, too. One study found that people with IBS miss an average of 13 workdays per year, costing the US around $20 billion in lost productivity.

Need for better treatment: Many people with IBS struggle to find treatments that work. This shows how important it is to keep researching IBS to understand it better and come up with better treatments.

Spreading the word: Because IBS is so common and affects life so much, we need to raise awareness, help people understand it, and encourage those suffering in silence to reach out for help and support.

IBS often flies under the radar and does not get treated well, which means a lot of people suffer without help. IBS is important to understand because it affects so many people and their lives. Diagnosing and treating IBS can be challenging and requires a team effort with medical, dietary, and mental health support. By raising awareness and understanding, healthcare professionals and people with IBS can work together to improve care. In addition, teaching everyone about IBS can reduce stigma and help people feel more empathy for those dealing with it.

Key takeaways:

- IBS is a disorder of gut-brain interaction (DGBI) that affects the small and large intestines, causing symptoms like abdominal pain, gas, bloating, and altered bowel habits.
- The history of IBS dates back to ancient civilizations. It has gone through various names and diagnostic criteria before being recognized as IBS in the mid-1900s.
- IBS affects around 10-15% of people in the US and is more common in women, with risk factors including age, family history, stress, and psychological factors.
- IBS can significantly impact daily life, including quality of life, social stigma, mental health, and economic burden, with healthcare costs estimated at $1.6 billion annually in the US alone.
- Raising awareness and understanding of IBS is essential to improve diagnosis and treatment, reduce stigma, and help those with IBS to reach out for help and support.

CHAPTER 2

Symptoms and Signs of Irritable Bowel Syndrome

"Life is like a box of chocolates; you never know what you're going to get"
- Forrest Gump

Amanda is a 35-year-old woman who came to see me recently with frequent abdominal pain and discomfort, bloating, and changes in bowel movements for about a year. She reported having loud noises in her belly at times, which can be quite embarrassing if she is in a meeting at work. Amanda also reported feeling fatigued and experiencing low energy, making it challenging to keep up with her job and daily activities. She has also been feeling anxious and depressed, which she believes is related to her IBS symptoms.

When I examined her, she had mild tenderness all over her abdomen. I did not feel any lumps or bumps. I ran some blood and stool tests which all came back normal. Based on her symptoms and excluding other causes of her symptoms, I diagnosed her with IBS. She was asked to follow a diet and prescribed medication to help manage her symptoms. Amanda also sought counseling to address her anxiety and depression.

Over time, Amanda could identify trigger foods and make dietary modifications that improved her symptoms. She also found that incorporating regular exercise and stress-reducing activities like yoga helped *with her fatigue and anxiety. With these strategies in place, Amanda was able to manage her IBS symptoms and improve her quality of life.*

Common Symptoms of IBS

IBS symptoms can vary a lot, but common symptoms include abdominal pain, changes in bowel movements, bloating, and gas. Interestingly, these symptoms mostly happen when we are awake and rarely when we are asleep. Other issues, like the feeling of incomplete evacuation of bowels, urgency, and mucus in the stool, are also symptoms of IBS. This chapter will explore these symptoms and how they affect people's lives.

Abdominal pain and discomfort

Abdominal pain is a key IBS symptom. People often feel a crampy or sharp pain in their lower abdomen, sometimes after eating. The pain might happen before or after going to the bathroom and could improve or persist after passing stool. For some, the pain is constant and interferes with daily life.

Changes in bowel movements

Changes in bowel movements, like diarrhea, constipation, or both, are common in IBS. People might feel an urgent need to go, struggle to go, or feel incomplete after going. Bowel movement frequency can also vary a lot.

Bloating and gas

Bloating and gas can be uncomfortable and embarrassing. This might be because of increased sensitivity to gas or changes in gut bacteria. Excessive belching or passing gas can make the situation worse.

A feeling of incomplete evacuation of bowels

This means you might still feel like you haven't fully emptied your bowels after using the restroom. It can be frustrating and leave you feeling uncomfortable throughout the day.

Urgency

Urgency refers to a sudden, strong need to use the restroom. This sensation can be quite distressing, as it might catch you off guard and require you to find a bathroom quickly.

Mucus in stool

Mucus is a slippery substance naturally found in the lining of your intestines. Sometimes, people with IBS may notice increased mucus in their stool. While this might sound alarming, it is usually not a cause for concern, as it can be a common symptom of IBS.

Physical Signs of IBS

Besides the above symptoms, some physical signs can be observed in people with IBS. Let's take a closer look at these physical signs.

1. **Abdominal tenderness:** One of the physical signs of IBS is abdominal tenderness, which means the stomach area might be sensitive or painful when pressed. This tenderness can result from gas and bloating, or it could be due to the heightened sensitivity of the gut, which is often seen in IBS sufferers. Remember that the location and intensity of tenderness vary from person to person and can fluctuate over time.

2. **Unusual bowel sounds:** Our digestive system is always at work, and it is common to hear some noises from the stomach,

especially when hungry or right after eating. However, these bowel sounds might be more noticeable and frequent in people with IBS. These sounds, sometimes called "borborygmi," can result from increased gas production or abnormal muscle contractions in the gut. Although these sounds can be a bit embarrassing, they are usually harmless.

3. **Bloating and swelling:** Another physical sign of IBS is bloating, where the abdominal area appears swollen or enlarged. This can be due to excess gas or irregular muscle contractions in the digestive tract. Bloating can cause discomfort and might even make it difficult to find clothes that fit comfortably.

4. **Altered stool appearance:** Although not a direct "physical sign," changes in stool appearance can indicate IBS. People with IBS might experience variations in stool consistency, ranging from hard, pellet-like stools to loose, watery bowel movements. The stool might also appear ribbon-like or have mucus present.

Associated Conditions of IBS

IBS can be linked to fatigue, low energy, anxiety, depression, and headaches, making life more challenging.

Fatigue and low energy

Many people with IBS experience fatigue and low energy levels. Some of the factors that contribute to this connection-

- **Chronic pain:** One reason for fatigue in IBS sufferers is the constant pain and discomfort they experience due to their condition. Dealing with chronic pain can be physically and mentally exhausting, making it difficult to stay energized throughout the day.

- **Changes in gut bacteria:** In people with IBS, changes in gut bacteria can lead to fatigue as the body struggles to maintain a healthy balance.
- **Avoiding physical activity:** Due to the pain and discomfort associated with IBS, some people might avoid physical activity for fear of aggravating their symptoms. However, a lack of exercise can contribute to feelings of fatigue and low energy.
- **Sleep disturbances:** IBS symptoms can cause sleep disturbances. Although IBS symptoms generally do not wake you up in the middle of the night, the symptoms may delay your bedtime. Poor sleep quality can lead to fatigue during the day.

Headaches and migraines

Headaches and migraines are often connected to IBS, but the exact link is still a mystery. Studies show that about 25% of IBS patients have migraines, while 18% have tension headaches. These numbers are lower in people who do not have IBS. Migraines and IBS share some features, like being more common in women and triggered by stress or anxiety. Both conditions also involve increased pain sensitivity and have specific foods that make symptoms worse.

Researchers have some theories about the cause of this link. One idea is that the gut-brain axis (*more on this later*) is involved in both conditions. Another possibility is that both involve issues in the central nervous system, especially with pain perception and processing. This could lead to overlapping symptoms like stomach pain and headaches.

Serotonin, a neurotransmitter that helps regulate pain and mood, might also play a role. Problems with serotonin signaling could contribute to IBS and migraines. Medications targeting serotonin receptors have been effective in treating both conditions.

Anxiety, depression, and IBS: a troubling trio

Anxiety and depression are common among people with IBS. Up to 60% of people with IBS deal with anxiety and up to 40% face depression. Constantly worrying about symptoms and their impact on daily life can increase anxiety, which can make symptoms worse. Depression may come from the burden IBS puts on everyday life, causing feelings of hopelessness and isolation.

The exact reasons behind this link are not fully understood, but the gut-brain axis is believed to play a part. Changes in the gut can affect the brain and vice versa. Stress, which can trigger IBS symptoms, may also lead to anxiety and depression. Additionally, changes in gut bacteria have been linked to both IBS and mental health disorders. Understanding the connection between IBS, anxiety, and depression is crucial for developing treatment plans that address IBS and related conditions like anxiety and depression.

Key takeaways:

- IBS symptoms include abdominal pain or discomfort, changes in bowel movements, bloating, and gas.
- Physical signs of IBS include abdominal tenderness, unusual bowel sounds, bloating and swelling, and altered stool appearance.
- Associated conditions of IBS include fatigue and low energy, headaches and migraines, anxiety, and depression.
- IBS-related fatigue can result from chronic pain, changes in gut bacteria, avoiding physical activity, and sleep disturbances.

- Headaches and migraines are often connected to IBS, possibly due to the gut-brain axis and pain perception and processing issues.
- Anxiety and depression are common among people with IBS, due to changes in the gut-brain axis and stress.

CHAPTER 3

Causes and Triggers of Irritable Bowel Syndrome

"Happiness is not a matter of intensity but of balance, order, rhythm, and harmony."
– Thomas Merton

The tangled web of IBS causes

IBS is a complex condition. The exact cause of IBS is not fully understood, but it is thought to be caused by many factors, including disturbance in the gut-brain axis, enteric nervous system (ENS) stimulation, visceral sensitivity, altered gut microbiome, immune system malfunction, and stress. In addition to these, several unknown factors may be playing a role in causing IBS or triggering IBS symptoms. Understanding the causes of IBS is crucial for correctly diagnosing and effectively managing symptoms.

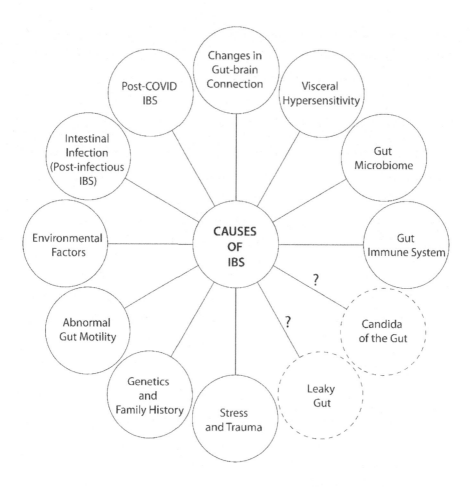

The gut-brain connection: a two-way street

Imagine your gut is like a radio, constantly sending and receiving signals. The gut-brain connection is a two-way communication channel between your belly and brain, allowing them to send messages back and forth. Sometimes, the signals get mixed up, and the way you feel emotionally can affect how your body physically responds.

In the 1950s, Dr. William H. Gantt, an American scientist, embarked on fascinating research using Pavlov's legendary dogs to explore the gut-brain connection. Ivan Pavlov, a Russian physiologist, had already established the concept of classical conditioning (e.g., Pavlov's dogs salivating at the sound of a bell) in dogs in the early 1900s. Gantt, who had worked with Pavlov, decided to apply these principles to understand the relationship between our bellies and brains.

Gantt performed rather unusual experiments on dogs by creating a tiny pouch in their stomachs. He then observed the dogs' reactions to various stimuli, like the sight or smell of food. Surprisingly, he found that when the dogs saw or smelled food, their stomachs produced gastric secretions, even if they didn't eat the food.

Things got even more interesting when Gantt discovered that the dogs' stomachs could be conditioned to respond to entirely unrelated stimuli, like the sound of a bell. This finding proved a strong connection between the brain, emotions, and the gut. Gantt's work also revealed that dogs could develop visceral hypersensitivity, making their guts more sensitive to stimuli after experiencing stress or trauma.

Thanks to Gantt's quirky experiments, we understand the intricate relationship between the gut and the brain, setting the stage for further research into the gut-brain axis and its impact on conditions like IBS.

The gut-brain axis communicates through neural, hormonal, and immunological pathways. The vagus nerve, a large nerve connecting the brain to the GI tract (digestive system), is a crucial neural communication route in the gut-brain axis. It sends signals from the brain to the enteric nervous system (ENS), influencing gut motility, secretion, and sensitivity.

Hormonal signals, such as those released by the hypothalamic-pituitary-adrenal (HPA) axis in response to stress, can also impact GI tract function. For example, cortisol, released by the adrenal glands when stressed, can affect immune cell activity in the GI tract and alter GI motility and secretion.

The gut-brain axis also includes immune cells in the central nervous system (CNS) and the GI tract. These cells produce signaling molecules that can affect the ENS and CNS functions and regulate the GI tract's immune response.

Enteric nervous system - the "brain" behind the gut feelings

Let's talk about the ENS, or as we like to call it, the "second brain" in your gut because it can operate independently from the central nervous system. Yep, you heard that right. You've got a brain in your gut! This gut-brain connection controls several physiological processes in the gastrointestinal system, including the secretion of digestive juices, modulation of immune function, and the movement of food through the digestive tract.

Your gut also signals your brain about hunger, fullness, and the need to use the bathroom. These signals come from the ENS. Remember those "butterflies in your stomach"? That's your ENS talking to you.

The term ENS was first introduced by the British neuroanatomist and neurophysiologist John Newport Langley in the late 19th century. The ENS is a complex network of over 500 million nerve cells that lines your entire digestive tract from your esophagus to your rectum. These nerve cells work together to control the entire digestive process, from breaking down food to absorbing nutrients and eliminating waste.

You might ask, "Why does my gut need its own brain? Doesn't my main brain already control everything?" Well, not exactly. While your main brain does play a role in regulating digestion through the gut-brain axis, the ENS is responsible for many of the automatic and unconscious processes that occur in your gut, like controlling the muscles that move food through the gut and regulating the secretion of digestive enzymes and hormones.

The gut has its own set of neurotransmitters, including serotonin, often called the "happy hormone." Changes in the levels of these neurotransmitters can lead to changes in mood and emotions. On the flip side, your brain can also send signals to your gut that affect how your digestive system functions. When you see, smell, or even think about food, your brain can send signals to your gut to produce digestive juices and prepare for a meal. That fresh smell of French fries making you hungry is the brain firing signals to your gut!

Let's say there's a miscommunication or a bad connection on this communication line. That's where things can get a little unstable. For example, suppose you're feeling anxious or stressed. Then your brain might send signals causing the gut to become overactive or underactive or cause you to feel pain in your gut. Similarly, your gut can send pain signals if something isn't feeling quite right. These changes can lead to the symptoms of IBS, like abdominal pain, bloating, and changes in bowel habits.

The enteric nervous system is a fascinating, complex, interconnected system that plays a vital role in our digestive health. By understanding how these systems work and interact with each other, we can better understand how to manage the symptoms of IBS and improve overall gut health. This emphasizes the importance of an integrated or holistic approach, focusing on both the physical and emotional aspects of IBS, which can result in more effective symptom management and improved quality of life.

Visceral hypersensitivity: when the gut gets too touchy

IBS can make your gut extra sensitive to the usual stuff like gas or food passing through, causing discomfort, pain, or bloating. This overreaction, called visceral hypersensitivity, is still a mystery. Genetics, gut bacteria changes, chronic stress, and enteric nervous system dysfunction might contribute to it.

Early-life stress plays a crucial role in IBS, as it can disrupt the gut-brain axis and exacerbate IBS symptoms. A 1998 study investigated the influence of early-life stress on IBS, revealing that individuals who experienced significant stress during World War II, such as bombings and food scarcity, had an increased likelihood of developing IBS later in life. This finding underscores the importance of stress as a potential cause of IBS.

In the 1930s, a Hungarian-Canadian scientist named Hans Selye, often called the "Father of Stress Research," conducted experiments on rats to explore the relationship between stress and gastrointestinal issues. Selye administered ovarian extracts to the rats and observed that their digestive systems exhibited strong reactions.

To further study this connection, Selye subjected the rats to various stressors, such as extreme temperatures, loud noises, and physical restraint. These stressful experiences provoked a similar response in the rats' digestive systems as the hormone injections. Selye named this response the "general adaptation syndrome," which involved the release of stress hormones like cortisol and adrenaline. His work significantly contributed to our understanding of how stress can negatively impact physical health, including the gastrointestinal system.

Selye's research on rats was groundbreaking and encouraged scientists to investigate the gut-brain connection and the sensitivity of our gastrointestinal systems. They found that stress can negatively affect our digestive system and impact how our brain responds to stress.

The gut microbiome – a tiny world in the gut

Our digestive system is home to countless microorganisms, including bacteria, viruses, and fungi, collectively known as the gut microbiome that aid in breaking down food, strengthening our immune system, and even influencing our brain function. These tiny helpers can affect how our gut functions, including movement, inflammation, and pain perception.

A healthy gut has a diverse community of microorganisms that work together. However, when this balance is disrupted, it can lead to a condition called dysbiosis, which has been associated with various health issues, including IBS.

People with IBS tend to have more bad bacteria than good ones compared to those without IBS. For example, one study in 2012 found that folks with IBS had fewer "good" bacteria like Bifidobacteria and Lactobacilli. Moreover, they had more of the not-so-great ones like Proteobacteria and Actinobacteria. These changes in gut bacteria can cause inflammation, changes in gut movement, and increased sensitivity—all things that play a part in IBS.

Stuff like stress, anxiety, infections, and antibiotics can affect the gut microbiome, leading to changes in gut function and even IBS. For example, astronauts who felt stressed and anxious during space missions had their gut microbiome go all weird, which affected their digestion.

Changes in the gut microbiome can also impact the brain and behavior, interfering with the gut-brain connection. Some experts think that gut bacteria might even influence our mood and mental health. In fact, some studies suggest a link between gut microbiome imbalance and issues like anxiety and depression.

The whole gut microbiome and IBS connection has totally changed how we see this complicated disorder. By learning more about how our gut microbiome affects our health, we can come up with better ways to prevent, manage, and treat IBS and other related problems.

The protector: the immune system and IBS

Our immune system is like our body's personal security guard, defending us from nasty stuff like bacteria, viruses, and other things that can make us sick. For people with IBS, though, their immune system can be a bit too jumpy, overreacting to small things. This super-sensitivity can lead to an over-the-top immune response and cause IBS symptoms.

Low-grade inflammation and immune cells gone wild

Studies indicate that individuals with IBS may experience a less severe type of inflammation that can still cause discomfort and aggravate IBS symptoms. This inflammation is associated with an increased number of immune cells, such as mast cells and T-cells, within the gut. These cells release histamine and cytokines (inflammation signals), leading to heightened sensitivity in the gut and the onset of IBS symptoms.

Gut barrier function and the immune system

The gut barrier is an essential component of the gastrointestinal tract, responsible for preventing harmful substances from entering the bloodstream while allowing nutrients to be absorbed. In one experiment, it was discovered that young rats that were separated from their mothers experienced a weakening of the gut lining, which is normally strengthened by mast cells during stressful situations. In some cases of IBS, stress can cause the gut barrier function to be compromised, allowing substances like bacteria and food particles to pass through the barrier and stimulate the immune system. This process, known as increased intestinal permeability or "leaky gut," can lead to an overactive immune response and contribute to IBS symptoms. *More on leaky gut later.*

The emotional connection: stress and trauma

Stress and emotions can play a significant role in IBS development and treatment. Stress makes our nervous system more sensitive to pain and gut issues, changing the way our brains and gut talk to each other.

Many studies have shown a link between early life traumas, stress, and IBS. For example, a 2011 study found that childhood trauma (like mental illness in the family, emotional abuse, or having an incarcerated family member) increased the risk of IBS later in life. Some studies show that a history of post-traumatic stress disorder can increase your odds of developing IBS by 3 to 4 times compared to others.

Dr. Bessel van der Kolk, a psychiatrist and expert on post-traumatic stress, has been digging deep into how trauma affects our brain and body and how painful experiences can impact our overall health. He's worked with many patients with rough pasts and noticed a pattern. In his book, "The Body Keeps the Score," he discusses the connection between trauma and health issues, including IBS. He's seen many cases where patients with a history of trauma ended up with IBS.

Let's look at different parts of brain involved in this communication and how they're affected by early life traumas:

- **Amygdala:** This little almond-shaped brain part handles emotions, especially fear, and anxiety. Trauma or stress can make it too active, messing with our gut signals.

- **Hippocampus:** Shaped like a seahorse, this brain region is vital for learning and memory. Trauma can mess with its function, causing our stress response to go off the rails and impact our gut.
- **Prefrontal Cortex:** This part of the brain makes decisions and controls our emotions. If it's not working well because of trauma, it can hurt our gut health.

Now, let's explore how early life traumas and past or present stress can lead to IBS:

- **HPA axis problems:** The HPA axis is our body's stress system. Bad experiences can make it go into overdrive, causing gut issues.
- **Gut bacteria changes:** Stress and trauma can mess with these bacteria, leading to IBS.
- **Leaky gut:** Stress can make the gut lining more permeable, letting stuff through too easily. This can cause inflammation and IBS symptoms.

Genetics and family history – inherited sensitivity

Having IBS in your family increases your chances of getting IBS. A study by the Mayo Clinic found that between 25% and 50% of IBS patients had at least one family member with the condition. Many genetic factors can play a part in developing IBS, like how your gut moves, inflammation, and how you feel pain. One gene that's been studied extensively is the serotonin transporter gene (SERT), which makes some people more likely to have IBS symptoms. When a person is healthy, serotonin is released into the gut and triggers an intestinal reflex. The SERT found in the gut wall cells removes the serotonin from the bowel. However, individuals with IBS have insufficient SERT, leading to an excess of serotonin in the gut which causes diarrhea. This excess serotonin also overloads the gut receptors, resulting in constipation.

There are other genes associated with immune function and gut motility that have been linked to IBS. However, genetic factors may only be applicable to certain IBS patients, and the extent to which genetics play a role in certain types of IBS may vary. Additionally, shared environmental factors such as lifestyle, diet, and stressors among family members can also contribute to the development of IBS.

Although genetics and family history may suggest the possibility of developing IBS, it is not a definite indicator. It is possible for individuals with a family history to never develop the condition, while those without a family history may still experience IBS.

Abnormal gut motility – when the gut loses its rhythm

Abnormal gut motility, or in other words, how the muscles in your intestines contract and move food, is thought to be a significant cause of IBS. Normally, these muscles work together to move food through your digestive system like a conveyor belt. But for people with IBS, these contractions can get out of whack, causing all kinds of symptoms.

Research shows that between 30% and 80% of IBS patients have weird gut motility. Using techniques like colonic manometry (a motility study), scientists have found that people with IBS often have stronger and more frequent colon contractions than those without IBS. This can make food move faster in the colon, leading to diarrhea.

Imaging studies, like MRI scans, have shown that people with IBS have slower food movement in the small intestine, which could cause bloating and stomach pain. It's not entirely clear why gut movement gets messed up in IBS, but stress, anxiety, certain foods, medications, and genetics might play a role in the issue.

The invisible enemy: environmental factors

Environmental factors, including toxins and pollution, might also contribute to developing and exacerbating IBS. Research has shown that exposure to pesticides or agricultural chemicals could elevate the risk of developing IBS. Additionally, air pollution has been reported to trigger symptoms in some individuals.

For instance, a study conducted in California in 2022 discovered a connection between exposure to particulate matter and airborne toxic releases from industrial facilities and increased IBS prevalence. Particulate matter includes tiny particles suspended in the air, which can be inhaled, causing health problems. Airborne toxic releases from facilities refer to discharging hazardous substances into the air, which can negatively affect human health.

These findings highlight the potential role of environmental pollution in IBS and suggest that reducing exposure to such pollution could help individuals better manage their IBS symptoms.

Intestinal infection and post-infectious IBS – when the gut doesn't heal

Gut infections can cause some damage and lead to IBS. Food poisoning or gastrointestinal infections have been tied to post-infectious IBS (PI-IBS), which makes up around 13% of all IBS cases.

PI-IBS can happen after a nasty bout of gastroenteritis caused by bacteria, viruses, or parasites. About 10% of patients might develop

IBS after a gastrointestinal infection, which can be tough to deal with and last for months or even years. Risk factors for PI-IBS include being female, being younger, feeling stressed during or before the infection, and the severity of the gut infection.

The connection between PI-IBS and infection really became known during the 2000 Walkerton water contamination incident, one of Canada's biggest water contamination disasters. The town's water supply got contaminated with E. coli and Campylobacter jejuni bacteria, causing over 2,300 people to get sick, 65 hospitalizations, and seven deaths. The tragedy was later blamed on a mix of heavy rainfall, contaminated wells, and lousy water treatment.

Within three years of this incident, about 28% of those who had gastrointestinal infections developed IBS symptoms. After eight years, 15% still had IBS symptoms, higher than those who weren't infected. This means that PI-IBS isn't necessarily a lifelong condition for everyone who had an infection since about half of PI-IBS patients got better over time.

The exact reasons for PI-IBS are still a bit of a mystery, but research suggests that the immune system might keep attacking the gut even after the initial infection is gone. In addition, harmful bacteria or viruses can alter the gut microbiome, resulting in inflammation and digestive problems. Interestingly, a 2023 study examined eight clinical trials that evaluated the efficacy of Mesalamine, a medication commonly used to treat intestinal inflammatory conditions like ulcerative colitis. The results of this study suggest that Mesalamine may be effective in treating IBS, indicating that IBS may involve mild inflammation of the gut that can be treated with medication.

Sarah:

One real-life story that illustrates the impact of PI-IBS involves a patient of mine named Sarah. Sarah was a healthy and active young woman in her early 40s when she traveled to Mexico for vacation. During her trip, she contracted severe food poisoning that left her bedridden for several days.

While Sarah eventually recovered from the initial infection, she continued to experience a range of gut-related symptoms for months afterward. She had frequent bouts of diarrhea, abdominal pain, and bloating. She found that many foods that she previously enjoyed now triggered uncomfortable symptoms.

When I saw Sarah, she had a lot of concerns- "Is this some parasite that I got while I was in Mexico, is this a bacterial infection, is it food poisoning that doesn't go away, is it colitis, or is it "all in my head"? She was desperate for answers. After running some blood tests, stool tests, and a colonoscopy, I diagnosed her with PI-IBS. While she was relieved to have a name for her condition, she was frustrated to learn that there was no quick fix for her symptoms.

She began working with me to develop a comprehensive treatment plan that included dietary modifications, probiotics, and counseling to address the anxiety and depression that accompanied her IBS. She's doing much better except for occasional flare-ups if she's not careful with certain foods.

Sarah's story is just one example of how PI-IBS can profoundly impact a person's life. While the exact mechanisms behind the condition are still being explored, researchers are making progress in understanding how infections can lead to long-term gut changes that contribute to the development of IBS.

The unexpected twist: post-COVID IBS

In the ongoing battle against COVID-19, an unexpected development has emerged: post-COVID IBS. This condition refers to starting or worsening IBS symptoms after a COVID-19 infection. The timeline for symptom development varies, and as research advances, we hope to understand this puzzling condition better.

The enigma: possible causes

The exact causes of post-COVID IBS are still a mystery, but several theories have surfaced:

1. **Gut-brain axis disruption:** COVID-19 might interrupt the communication between the gut and brain, leading to IBS symptoms.
2. **Direct viral effects:** The virus could directly harm the digestive system, causing inflammation and gut lining damage, which may contribute to IBS symptoms.
3. **Altered gut microbiome:** COVID-19 might disturb the balance of bacteria in the gut, leading to IBS symptoms.
4. **Immune system response:** The body's response to the virus could trigger or worsen IBS symptoms.

Symptoms:

Post-COVID IBS symptoms resemble typical IBS symptoms, including:

- Abdominal pain or cramping
- Bloating and gas
- More people develop IBS-D compared to other types of IBS (IBS-C, IBS-M, and IBS-U)
- Mucus in the stool
- The urgency to have a bowel movement

These symptoms can vary from person to person and may change over time.

The key differences: post-COVID IBS vs. regular IBS and PI-IBS

Post-COVID IBS, regular IBS, and PI-IBS share similarities, but there are important differences:

1. **Onset:** Post-COVID IBS starts or worsens after a COVID-19 infection, while regular IBS has various triggers. PI-IBS arises after acute gastroenteritis caused by bacteria, non-COVID-19 viruses, or parasites.
2. **Immune system involvement:** The immune response to COVID-19 might play a more prominent role in post-COVID IBS than in regular IBS or PI-IBS.
3. **Duration:** The duration of symptoms may differ between the three conditions. It's unclear whether post-COVID IBS symptoms will persist long-term or eventually resolve on their own.

The path to recovery: treatment options

Treating post-COVID IBS is pretty much like treating regular IBS. But it is critical to chat with your healthcare provider about any left-over COVID-19 effects, as they might recommend extra treatments or check-ups.

The road ahead

Post-COVID IBS is another hurdle for people recovering from COVID-19. Our understanding of the condition will improve as we learn more through ongoing research. In the meantime, folks with post-COVID IBS symptoms need to team up with healthcare professionals to create personalized treatment plans. By tackling the unique aspects of post-COVID IBS, we can help those affected get their lives back on track and enjoy a better quality of life.

Leaky gut and IBS: a tale of a mysterious condition

Picture your gut as a brick wall, with cells as bricks and tight bonds called "tight junctions" as the mortar. This wall is like your body's superhero, letting in the good stuff (nutrients) while keeping out the bad stuff (toxins). But sometimes, this wall gets a bit leaky, and that's when issues begin.

Leaky gut syndrome, or increased intestinal permeability, is a hot debate. While still controversial, evidence hints that it might play a part in conditions like inflammatory bowel disease (IBD), celiac disease, and autoimmune disorders. For example, a 2021 study found that IBD patients had lower levels of a protein called ZO-1, which helps keep the gut wall strong. This finding suggests that ZO-1 could be a potential target for treating these inflammatory conditions.

But what's leaky gut's role in IBS? It's kind of up in the air. Some studies claim IBS patients have a leakier gut than healthy folks, which could lead to symptoms like abdominal pain and bloating. However, other studies don't agree.

Despite the uncertainty, there is some proof that diet and lifestyle factors might contribute to leaky gut and worsen IBS symptoms. This idea could be especially relevant for patients with PI-IBS, where the gut lining gets damaged, letting bacteria and toxins sneak in, triggering immune responses, and causing symptoms like pain and diarrhea.

In short, a leaky gut might not be the main bad guy in IBS, but keeping your gut wall strong is important for overall health. Eating a balanced diet, managing stress, and avoiding harmful substances can shield your body from toxins and lower the risk of developing gut-related health issues.

The Candida conundrum: Is Candida of the gut really the cause of gut problems?

Many people believe that Candida, a yeast called Candida albicans, is responsible for various gut problems, including IBS. They often come to me with stool microbiome test results and a self-diagnosis of "candida overgrowth" obtained from Dr. Google to support this theory. However, are these tests and claims trustworthy? Let's examine the issue more closely.

Candida is a type of yeast that naturally occurs in our bodies, particularly in the gut. In small amounts, it is harmless, but when it grows out of control, it can cause bloating and digestive issues. Some practitioners believe that this overgrowth can damage the gut lining and cause inflammation and IBS symptoms. However, research does not entirely support this idea.

Stool microbiome tests that claim to reveal your gut's microbiome may not be as reliable as you would expect. One significant problem is that these tests have random reference ranges that differ between labs. There is not enough research to determine what normal Candida levels should be, resulting in confusion and frustration.

Many studies have investigated the potential relationship between Candida overgrowth and IBS, but the results are all over the place. Some show a higher prevalence of Candida colonization in IBS patients. In contrast, others find no significant difference compared to healthy individuals.

The relationship between Candida overgrowth and IBS is complex and not yet fully understood. Experts suggest focusing on other factors like diet, stress, and an altered gut microbiome rather than solely blaming Candida overgrowth.

In conclusion, scientific evidence does not strongly support the notion that systemic Candida overgrowth causes IBS. However, since some evidence suggests that Candida overgrowth may contribute to gut issues, it may be worth considering an anti-Candida diet as a last resort. *More on the anti-candida diet in Chapter 6.*

The food factor: how diet plays a role in IBS

Food sensitivities and intolerances

Food sensitivities and intolerances are not as severe as allergies, but knowing which foods trigger symptoms is important for managing IBS. About 70% of people with IBS have food sensitivities or intolerances, which can lead to bloating, gas, and diarrhea or even cause gut inflammation, making IBS symptoms worse.

Lactose intolerance is a common IBS-related issue where people cannot digest lactose found in dairy products. Lactose intolerance is different from IBS, but it can worsen symptoms if you have both.

Gluten sensitivity is another big one. Gluten, a protein in wheat, barley, and rye, can trigger immune responses in those with celiac disease, damaging the small intestine and causing various symptoms. While only a small percentage of IBS sufferers have celiac disease, a gluten-free diet might help some.

FODMAPs (Fermentable **O**ligosaccharides, **D**isaccharides, **M**onosaccharides, and **P**olyols) are found in many foods. They can cause digestive trouble for some with IBS. A low-FODMAP diet has been a game-changer for many IBS patients.

Trigger foods

Other IBS triggers include high-fat foods, caffeine, alcohol, fizzy drinks, chocolate, artificial sweeteners, spicy foods, and histamine-rich foods (like certain fish, veggies, wine, beer, and fermented foods).

Dietary changes can ease IBS symptoms, but what works for one person might not work for another. Healthcare professionals might suggest an elimination diet to find your specific triggers. Keeping a food diary can be a huge help for tracking symptoms and avoiding problem foods. *See Chapter 6 for more information.*

The curious link between hormones and IBS

The endocrine system sends out hormones, which act like chemical text messages to control different bodily functions, including digestion. Women are more susceptible to IBS, and their symptoms can vary during their menstrual cycle, pregnancy, or menopause.

Here's how hormones can impact IBS symptoms:

- **Altered gut motility:** Hormones like serotonin and cortisol can affect how fast or slow food travels through your digestive system. Imbalances can lead to constipation (slow transit) or diarrhea (rapid transit). For example, cortisol, the stress hormone, can trigger serotonin release, potentially causing diarrhea in some people with IBS.
- **Changing pain sensitivity:** Hormones like estrogen and progesterone can alter how you feel pain signals in your gut, leading to more discomfort during IBS flare-ups. Estrogen tends to increase pain sensitivity, while progesterone has the opposite effect.

The monthly cycle and its impact on IBS

Female hormones, estrogen, and progesterone go up and down throughout the menstrual cycle. As estrogen levels rise and fall, and progesterone levels increase and stay high until the next cycle begins, these hormonal shifts can affect IBS symptoms. These changes can impact gut function and pain sensitivity, worsening IBS symptoms before or during periods.

Pregnancy and IBS

Pregnancy brings many hormonal changes that help the baby grow but can also majorly affect a woman's gut. Hormones like estrogen and progesterone can relax the muscles in the GI tract, slowing down food movement and causing constipation, bloating, and tummy discomfort—classic IBS symptoms.

But constipation is not the only issue during pregnancy. Some women might also have diarrhea or fluctuating bowel habits, making IBS management trickier. In addition, stress, a common pregnancy factor, can worsen IBS symptoms.

Menopause

During menopause, hormone levels drop, which can influence IBS symptoms. Some women might see an improvement, while others could find their symptoms more unpredictable. Lower estrogen levels can also weaken the pelvic floor, leading to constipation or incontinence.

Key takeaways:

- IBS causes are multifaceted, including gut-brain interaction, enteric nervous system, visceral hypersensitivity, gut microbiome imbalances, immune system activation, inflammation, and altered gut motility.
- Stress and previous emotional trauma can exacerbate IBS symptoms.
- Genetic factors and family history may influence your likelihood of developing IBS.
- Potential links between environmental factors, such as toxins and pollution, and IBS are being explored.
- Post-infectious IBS may emerge following gastrointestinal infections.
- The prevalence of post-COVID IBS is a rising concern.
- While leaky gut and Candida overgrowth are not primary causes of IBS, they may still contribute to the condition.
- Food sensitivities, intolerances, and specific trigger foods can aggravate IBS symptoms.
- Hormonal fluctuations, experienced during menstruation, pregnancy, and menopause, can impact IBS symptoms.

CHAPTER 4

Diagnosis of Irritable Bowel Syndrome

"Medicine is a science of uncertainty and an art of probability."
– Sir William Osler

Cracking the IBS code: an overview of the diagnostic process for IBS

Diagnosing IBS can be quite challenging. Unlike a urinary tract infection which can be easily detected through a simple urine test, diagnosing IBS is a more complex and sometimes confusing process. This is because IBS involves a combination of symptoms and lacks a specific diagnostic test. In such cases, healthcare professionals rely on established criteria or a checklist to determine if an individual exhibits all the necessary signs and symptoms associated with the condition.

The Rome Criteria

The Rome Criteria were established in 1989 when a group of gastro-enterologists met in Rome (hence the name) to create guidelines for diagnosing IBS. The Rome I Criteria focused on abdominal pain or discomfort lasting at least 12 weeks in the previous year, along with two or more symptoms: pain relief with bowel movement, onset associated with a change in stool frequency, or onset associated with a change in stool form.

But the Rome I Criteria were not perfect, so they evolved as more research on IBS was conducted. In 1999, the Rome II Criteria added new symptoms like bloating and incomplete evacuation while refining diagnostic criteria for constipation-predominant and diarrhea-predominant IBS.

Rome III Criteria arrived in 2006, providing even more specific diagnostic criteria. They included eliminating red-flag symptoms that might suggest another diagnosis.

The Rome IV Criteria, which were introduced in 2016, further refined the diagnostic categories for IBS, providing clinicians with a more comprehensive guide.

According to these criteria, IBS is characterized by recurrent abdominal pain or discomfort occurring at least **one day a week** for a **minimum of 3 months**, accompanied by **two or more** of the following symptoms:

1. Pain related to defecation: Pain is alleviated by defecation, or its onset is associated with a change in stool frequency.
2. Changes in stool frequency: Symptoms are connected to variations in the number of bowel movements.
3. Changes in stool form or appearance: Symptoms are associated with alterations in stool consistency or appearance.

Different Types of IBS

The Rome IV criteria also classify IBS into four subtypes based on the patient's predominant bowel habit:

1. **IBS with diarrhea (IBS-D):** Patients experience recurrent abdominal pain or discomfort and diarrhea symptoms.

2. **IBS with constipation (IBS-C):** Patients experience recurrent abdominal pain or discomfort and constipation symptoms.

3. **Mixed IBS (IBS-M):** Patients experience recurrent abdominal pain or discomfort and both constipation and diarrhea symptoms.

4. **IBS unclassified (IBS-U):** Patients meet diagnostic criteria for IBS but cannot be accurately categorized into one of the other three subtypes.

The prevalence of each subtype may vary depending on the population being studied, but the approximate percentages for the IBS subtypes are as follows:

- IBS-D: 40% of IBS patients
- IBS-C: 35% of IBS patients
- IBS-M: 20% of IBS patients
- IBS-U: 5% of IBS patients

The Rome IV Criteria stress that diagnosing IBS needs a complete look at the patient's symptoms and medical history. IBS used to be a "diagnosis of exclusion," – meaning it is diagnosed by ruling out other causes. But the current approach emphasizes that not all patients need a battery of tests before confirming the diagnosis. IBS can be diagnosed based on symptoms alone, particularly for patients under 40 without any alarming or "red flag symptoms". This means that excessive testing is unnecessary.

Diagnosing IBS is tricky, but with the Rome Criteria and a thorough check of symptoms and medical history, healthcare providers can give an accurate diagnosis and the right treatment plan. If you have IBS symptoms, you must tell your healthcare provider everything about your symptoms and medical history to help in the diagnostic process.

Watch out for red-flag symptoms

When exploring IBS, particular "red flag" symptoms might signal a more serious issue and require extra attention. These symptoms include:

- Blood in your stool or rectal bleeding
- Anemia (low red blood cell count)
- Losing weight without trying
- A family history of colon cancer
- Symptoms appearing after age 50
- Nighttime symptoms that disrupt sleep
- Ongoing diarrhea that doesn't improve with over-the-counter medications
- Abdominal pain that is not relieved by passing gas or having a bowel movement
- New symptoms appearing in someone who was previously symptom-free
- Symptoms that keep getting worse over time.

It is important to address any red flags related to your digestive health with your healthcare provider. They may suggest additional tests or refer you to a gastroenterologist for further evaluation.

It is worth noting that while these symptoms can be concerning, they don't always indicate a serious issue and can often be managed with proper treatment. If you don't have any alarm symptoms, your provider may start treatment without further testing. However, in some cases, you might need more tests like imaging or colonoscopy to rule out other potential causes of digestive problems.

The power of communication

To get the best care possible, your healthcare provider needs to know the following:

- How your symptoms began (suddenly or gradually)
- How long they have been going on (short-term or long-term)
- The location and nature of the pain (constant or intermittent)
- Any other symptoms (like bloating or changes in bowel movements)
- Foods that trigger your symptoms
- Medications you are taking and if symptoms started after starting certain medications
- Family history of digestive problems, including inflammatory bowel disease, celiac disease, lactose intolerance, and IBS
- Any history of abuse or trauma
- Prior diagnosis of anxiety or depression

Diagnostic tests

In addition to a thorough medical history and physical exam, doctors use various tests to help rule out other potential causes of your symptoms. Here are some of the tests that may be used in the IBS diagnostic process:

1. **Blood tests:** These tests help rule out conditions like celiac disease, inflammatory bowel disease, thyroid problems, and anemia. Some standard tests include a complete blood count, a complete metabolic panel, C-reactive protein, thyroid function tests, and a celiac disease test.
2. **Stool tests:** These check for infection, inflammation, or blood in the stool. They look for a biomarker called fecal calprotectin

and check for infections like parasites or certain bacteria causing gastrointestinal issues.

3. **Imaging studies:** Tests like an abdominal ultrasound, CT scan, or MRI help check for abnormalities in abdominal organs such as the liver, pancreas, or gallbladder.

4. **Colonoscopy:** This procedure allows doctors to examine the inside of the large intestine using a flexible tube with a camera. It helps spot inflammation, ulcers, polyps, or tumors that might cause IBS-like symptoms. Patients need to follow a special diet and bowel prep before the procedure.

5. **Upper endoscopy:** In this procedure, a small camera is passed through the mouth to examine the digestive tract. Upper endoscopy evaluates the esophagus, stomach, and duodenum. This procedure helps detect inflammation, ulcers, and other abnormalities like celiac disease.

6. **Other diagnostic tests:** Breath tests can diagnose conditions that cause IBS-like symptoms. For example, a lactose intolerance breath test detects lactose intolerance, which can cause bloating, gas, and diarrhea. A breath test for SIBO diagnoses this condition, which can also cause IBS-like symptoms.

Remember, not all these tests will be necessary for everyone with IBS-like symptoms. The specific tests will depend on several factors, including your medical history, symptoms, and physical exam. Your healthcare provider will work with you to determine the most appropriate tests to diagnose or rule out other conditions before confirming an IBS diagnosis. In some cases, IBS might be diagnosed based on your symptoms alone, without the need for extensive testing.

Medical conditions that mimic or overlap with IBS

Celiac disease

Celiac disease and IBS both cause digestive issues, but they have different underlying causes. Celiac disease is an autoimmune disorder triggered by gluten, a protein in wheat, barley, and rye. Although someone with IBS may also have celiac disease, having one condition does not necessarily mean it causes the other. Studies say up to 4% of IBS patients might also have celiac disease.

The main difference is that celiac disease damages the small intestine's lining, affecting nutrient absorption. IBS, however, does not cause physical damage to the digestive system.

If you suspect that you may have celiac disease, tests are available, including a blood test to check for gluten antibodies and a small intestine biopsy for confirmation. It is important to note that these tests require consuming gluten, so if you are following a gluten-free diet, you will need to reintroduce gluten before getting tested.

Inflammatory bowel disease

IBS and inflammatory bowel disease (IBD) can both cause belly pain, bloating, and change in bowel movements. But there are some hints to help tell them apart. With IBS, the pain and discomfort usually go away after a bowel movement. There is often a change in bowel habits, like constipation, diarrhea, or a mix of both. IBS does not cause damage to the lining of the bowel, and there are no signs of inflammation in blood or stool tests.

In contrast, IBD causes more severe symptoms like bloody or mucus-filled diarrhea, weight loss, and fever. The pain and discomfort often stick around even after bowel movements. IBD can cause structural changes to the bowel, seen in imaging studies like CT scans or colonoscopies. Patients with IBD often have elevated inflammatory markers in their blood and stool.

Differentiating between the two is crucial as the treatment methods vary. IBD needs a more aggressive approach, using medications to calm the immune system and reduce bowel inflammation.

Diverticulitis

Although Diverticulitis and IBS share some similarities, they are distinct conditions. Diverticulitis is characterized by inflammation or infection of the small pouches (diverticula) in the colon's wall. The pain associated with this condition is sudden and sharp, and typically felt on the lower left side of the abdomen. In some cases, the pain can be intense and accompanied by fever or chills and may require antibiotics or even hospitalization. In contrast, IBS pain is chronic and ongoing.

IBS vs. colon cancer: the hidden enemy

While IBS can be a bothersome condition, it does not seriously threaten your health. In contrast, colon cancer is a dangerous condition that can be life-threatening if not detected early. Symptoms of colon cancer may include belly pain and bloating, ongoing changes in bowel movements, like diarrhea or constipation, and blood in the stool.

Blood in the stool is the giveaway sign that sets colon cancer apart from IBS. This can be a red flag for colon cancer, especially if it is persistent and unexplained. Not all colon cancer cases have blood in the stool, but it is a common symptom. Other hints include unexplained weight loss, fatigue, and weakness.

Colon cancer needs quick action, with treatments like surgery or chemo, to beat cancer and stop it from spreading. If you notice changes in bowel movements, abdominal pain, or blood in the stool, don't wait – talk to your healthcare provider.

Functional dyspepsia: the upper GI Cousin of IBS

Functional dyspepsia (FD) and IBS might feel like they are similar, with overlapping symptoms and similar causes, but they have fundamental differences. The main difference is where they hit. IBS goes for the lower digestive tract, while FD targets the upper part. I like to call FD as "upper GI cousin" of IBS. FD symptoms include upper belly pain, bloating, nausea, and feeling full after eating just a small amount of food. The exact cause is still a mystery, but it could be due to gut motility issues, increased sensitivity, and disordered brain-gut signals.

The Rome criteria, like with IBS, are used to diagnose FD. Rome IV criteria for FD include one or more symptoms like feeling full quickly after eating, upper belly pain, or burning – with no other explanation. Symptoms must be around for at least three months and have started six months before diagnosis. Tests for FD may include upper GI endoscopy, gastric emptying scan, lactose intolerance testing, hydrogen breath testing, and tests for H. pylori infection.

FD and IBS can coexist, with one condition that may be setting you up for the other. Research shows that 35%-40% of IBS patients may also have FD, and FD sufferers are more likely to have IBS symptoms.

Treatment for FD and IBS often involves similar strategies, like lifestyle changes, diet changes, and medications. Antidepressants, cognitive-behavioral therapy, and proton pump inhibitors or prokinetic agents may help some people with FD.

In short, IBS and FD are different but related. They share some symptoms but differ in where they strike and how they are diagnosed.

Lactose intolerance: the dairy dilemma

Lactose intolerance is when you cannot break down lactose, a sugar in milk and dairy because your small intestine does not have enough of an enzyme called lactase. When lactose is not digested right, it can lead to bloating, gas, diarrhea, and belly pain. Remember, lactose intolerance is not a milk allergy which is an immune reaction to milk proteins and can cause more severe symptoms like hives, wheezing, and anaphylaxis.

Lactose intolerance and IBS may look alike, but they are different. However, IBS patients might be more likely to become lactose intolerant. Also, lactose intolerant people might have IBS-like symptoms without actually having IBS.

Lactose intolerance is pretty common, affecting around 75% of the world's population at least to some extent. In the US, up to 30 million adults are lactose intolerant. It is more common among African Americans, Hispanic and Asian Americans and less common in people of European descent. As we get older, our chances of becoming lactose intolerant increase because lactase production goes down.

To know if you are lactose intolerant, you can get tested. One popular test is the hydrogen breath test – you drink a lactose drink and measure the hydrogen in your breath over a few hours. If lactose is not digested, bacteria in your large intestine break it down, creating hydrogen gas that you breathe out.

Small Intestinal Bacterial Overgrowth (SIBO)

SIBO is a condition where bacteria overgrow in the small intestine, which usually has low levels of bacteria. Large intestine bacteria infiltrate the small intestine during SIBO, upsetting its balance. Symptoms of SIBO and IBS may be similar, such as bloating, stomach pain, diarrhea, and constipation. Excess bacteria in your small intestine break down food and produce gas and other substances that irritate your gut, causing discomfort.

IBS and SIBO are two separate conditions that are closely related and often occur together. Some studies found that up to 78% of people with IBS could have SIBO. Although they cause similar symptoms, it is important to understand that they are distinct conditions. Research suggests that SIBO may contribute to the onset or worsening of IBS symptoms for some individuals, but the relationship between the two can be confusing.

Factors that can lead to SIBO include:

- **Slow gut motility:** If your small intestine's muscles are not working right, food takes too long to move through your gut, giving bacteria a chance to overgrow.
- **Low stomach acid:** Stomach acid helps kill bacteria that enter your stomach. If you do not have enough acid, bacteria can survive and sneak into your small intestine.
- **Structural issues:** Physical blockages or prior surgery of your small intestine can create a stagnant environment that is perfect for bacteria to thrive.
- **Weak immune system:** A weakened immune system can make it more difficult for your body to control bacterial growth in

the gut, leading to an imbalance and potential overgrowth of harmful bacteria.

- **Changes in your gut's bacterial balance:** The gut's natural bacterial balance, or microbiome, is essential for maintaining overall gut health. Disruptions to this balance, caused by factors such as poor diet, stress, or antibiotic use, can lead to the overgrowth of harmful bacteria and contribute to gut-related issues, including SIBO and IBS.

To diagnose SIBO, your doctor might recommend a hydrogen breath test. You will drink a solution with lactulose or glucose, and they will check the levels of hydrogen and methane in your breath at different times. If these levels are high, it could mean you may have SIBO. Treating SIBO sometimes can help improve IBS symptoms too. However, working with your healthcare provider to find the proper treatment for your situation is essential.

Treating SIBO involves:

- **Antibiotics:** Taking antibiotics, like rifaximin (Xifaxan), can help lower the number of bacteria in your small intestine, giving you relief from bloating and other symptoms.
- **Dietary changes:** Some diets, like the low-FODMAP diet or the specific carbohydrate diet, can help you manage SIBO-related bloating by limiting the carbs that bacteria love to consume. Make sure to follow these diets with a healthcare provider or a registered dietitian's guidance.
- **Probiotics:** We're still exploring how probiotics can help with SIBO. Some studies show that certain strains might help balance gut bacteria and improve symptoms.

- **Motility agents:** If a slow-moving gut causes SIBO, your doctor might prescribe medications to speed things up and prevent SIBO from returning.
- **Lifestyle changes:** Regular exercise, stress management, and good sleep can all help create a healthier gut and keep SIBO from coming back.

In short, there is a strong connection between SIBO and IBS. If you have IBS and your symptoms don't improve with other treatments, it is essential to check for SIBO. With the correct diagnosis and treatment, many people with SIBO and IBS can see significant improvements in their symptoms.

SID: the sugar-breaking struggle

Sucrase-Isomaltase Deficiency (SID) is a rare genetic disorder that affects the digestive system's ability to break down specific sugars such as sucrose and maltose. It is also known as sucrose galactase deficiency.

Sucrase-isomaltase is an enzyme that is produced in the small intestine and plays a crucial role in breaking down complex sugars into simpler forms that the body can absorb. Individuals with SID do not produce enough of this enzyme, which leads to incomplete digestion of sucrose and starches. Inability to fully digest these foods can cause symptoms such as diarrhea, gas, bloating, and belly pain after consuming sugar-containing foods (like white table sugar) or starchy foods (like bread, cookies, crackers, and potatoes).

SID symptoms usually appear in infancy, soon after babies begin consuming solid foods containing sucrose or other complex sugars. Common symptoms include bloating, belly pain, diarrhea, and failure to thrive. Severe cases may lead to malnutrition and dehydration.

Doctors diagnose SID using a non-invasive breath test. The patient drinks a solution containing a specific amount of sugar (usually sucrose), and if hydrogen and/or methane levels in the breath samples increase, it indicates undigested sugar has reached the large intestine and is being fermented by bacteria - a sign of SID. However, this test is not commonly used and is not the preferred diagnostic tool. Doctors typically base their diagnosis on symptoms, family history, and genetic testing.

To treat SID, patients must avoid foods with complex sugars like sucrose and maltose. Instead, they should consume carbs from alternative sources such as glucose and fructose. Enzyme products like Sucraid, which contains the enzyme sucrase, can help patients digest and absorb carbs more effectively. This medication is available by prescription and is an effective treatment for SID.

Fibromyalgia: unraveling the mystery and its IBS connection

Let's dive into fibromyalgia, a puzzling and sometimes misunderstood condition. Fibromyalgia is a chronic disorder that causes widespread pain, tenderness, throughout your body and fatigue. It can also lead to sleep problems, mood swings, and cognitive difficulties, making daily tasks challenging. The catch? There is no specific test for fibromyalgia, so doctors diagnose it by evaluating symptoms and ruling out other conditions.

Fibromyalgia's exact cause remains a mystery, but experts think it entails a mix of genetic, environmental, and psychological factors.

Some theories point to an overactive nervous system, hormonal imbalances, or an unusual stress response.

Interestingly, fibromyalgia and IBS seem to be linked. One study showed that up to 32% of people with IBS also had fibromyalgia, and 49% of those with fibromyalgia also had IBS. Another study from England showed an even closer relationship - up to 70% of fibromyalgia patients also have IBS and 65% of IBS patients experience fibromyalgia symptoms.

Despite having different symptoms, these conditions share some features, which may explain why they often happen together.

- **Overlapping causes:** Both fibromyalgia and IBS involve increased pain sensitivity. People with either condition may feel discomfort more strongly than those without.
- **Common triggers:** Stress and anxiety can make both fibromyalgia and IBS symptoms worse. Managing stress is vital to treating both conditions.
- **Shared biological mechanisms:** Some researchers think that fibromyalgia and IBS might share similar underlying mechanisms, like altered pain processing in the central nervous system, dysfunction in the autonomic nervous system, or low-grade inflammation.

If you are grappling with IBS and fibromyalgia, fear not – there are ways to manage them simultaneously.

Some strategies to help you cope:

- **Medication:** Certain medications, like some antidepressants, can ease IBS and fibromyalgia symptoms. Consult your healthcare provider to determine the best medication plan for you.

- **Diet and nutrition:** A well-balanced diet can benefit IBS and fibromyalgia symptoms. Consider collaborating with a dietitian to develop a personalized meal plan that accounts for IBS-related dietary restrictions.
- **Exercise:** Regular low-impact exercises, such as walking, swimming, or yoga, can alleviate pain and fatigue in both conditions. It can boost your mood and overall well-being.
- **Stress management:** Mastering stress management techniques is crucial since stress can worsen IBS and fibromyalgia symptoms. Experiment with mindfulness meditation, deep breathing exercises, or progressive muscle relaxation to keep stress under control.
- **Sleep hygiene:** Enhancing sleep quality can significantly impact IBS and fibromyalgia symptoms. Stick to a consistent sleep schedule, establish a calming bedtime routine, and create a comfortable, sleep-friendly environment.
- **Professional Support:** A team of healthcare professionals – including doctors, therapists, and dietitians – can help you tackle the complexities of managing IBS and fibromyalgia, providing guidance, support, and essential tools to improve your quality of life.

CFS and IBS: double trouble

Chronic Fatigue Syndrome (CFS) is when extreme tiredness does not go away with rest. Interestingly, there is a link between IBS and CFS, with many people with IBS also dealing with chronic fatigue.

Studies show that around 35% to 90% of people with CFS also have IBS. The range is broad because different studies use different methods and diagnostic criteria. Conversely, around 10% to 20% of people with IBS suffer from CFS.

The exact reason for this overlap is a mystery, but researchers think shared factors like immune system issues, psychological factors, gut microbiome imbalances, and central nervous system problems might play a role in both conditions. Treating CFS and IBS usually involves medications, cognitive-behavioral therapy, and lifestyle changes.

IBS in kids: more than just grown-up troubles

IBS is not just for grown-ups. Kids and teenagers can also deal with this tummy turmoil, which is one of the most common digestive problems they face.

IBS symptoms in the young

Kids with IBS can have symptoms like adults, such as stomach pain, bloating, diarrhea, constipation, and changes in bowel movements. These symptoms can mess with their daily lives, affecting school attendance and their ability to enjoy everyday activities.

Diagnosing IBS in kids

Figuring out if a kid has IBS can be tricky. Little ones might have difficulty describing their symptoms, while older ones might feel too embarrassed or shy to discuss them. Doctors often count on parents' observations to better understand the child's situation.

Ruling out other troublemakers

Not all kids with tummy troubles have IBS. Doctors must rule out other conditions like inflammatory bowel disease, celiac disease, food allergies, lactose intolerance, acid reflux, and functional dyspepsia. Kids are also more likely to have functional constipation or abdominal pain, which can look like IBS. A thorough medical evaluation and tests are essential to determine the real issue.

What makes diagnosing IBS in kids special

IBS can show up differently in kids compared to adults. For example, kids with IBS might be more sensitive to certain foods like dairy or gluten. They may also experience diarrhea and vomiting more often, while adults usually deal with constipation and bloating. Stress related to school or social situations could also set off IBS symptoms in kids.

Another key difference is that kids with IBS may face more emotional and psychological challenges related to their condition, like anxiety or depression.

In a nutshell, IBS can affect kids and teenagers, needing extra care and attention when diagnosing and treating them. The approach to treating IBS in kids might differ from adults, considering their unique symptoms and potential effects on growth and development. Keeping a close eye on their progress and adjusting treatment as needed, with the help of a pediatrician or gastroenterologist, is vital for managing their tummy troubles.

When should you consult a doctor for IBS symptoms?

If you are dealing with IBS symptoms, you might be thinking about when to see a doctor. While many people manage their IBS with lifestyle changes, some situations require medical attention.

Watch out for these warning signs

Although IBS is typically not life-threatening, certain warning signs could point to a more serious condition. Consult a doctor if you notice any of the following:

- **Rectal bleeding or blood in your stool:** This could suggest inflammatory bowel disease (IBD) or colon cancer.
- **Severe or constant abdominal pain:** This might indicate a bowel obstruction or infection.
- **Unexplained weight loss:** This could signal cancer or malabsorption.
- **Difficulty swallowing:** This might suggest an esophageal disorder or cancer.
- **Anemia:** This could indicate bleeding in the digestive tract.

When to seek medical help

If your IBS symptoms impact your daily life, seeking medical help is essential. Some symptoms that may require medical attention include:

- **Frequent diarrhea or constipation:** See a doctor if you have more than three bowel movements per day or fewer than three per week.
- **Abdominal pain or discomfort:** If pain or discomfort doesn't improve after a bowel movement or dietary changes, consult a doctor.
- **Persistent bloating or gas:** If bloating or gas doesn't improve with dietary or lifestyle changes, see a doctor.
- **Changes in bowel habits:** If you observe changes in your stool's shape or consistency, consult a doctor.
- **Symptoms interfering with daily life:** Discuss treatment options with your doctor if IBS symptoms affect your daily activities.
- **Family history:** If your family has a history of inflammatory bowel disease or colon cancer, talk to your doctor about your risk and any recommended screenings.

To sum up, if your IBS symptoms mess with your daily life or make you worried, it is imperative to see a doctor. They can help determine the cause of your symptoms and develop a treatment plan to manage them and improve your life.

Key takeaways:

- Diagnosing IBS can be complex, as it involves a combination of symptoms.
- The Rome IV criteria aid in identifying IBS, taking into account recurrent abdominal pain/discomfort, alterations in stool frequency/form, and relief after bowel movements.
- IBS has four subtypes: IBS-C, IBS-D, IBS-M, and IBS-U.
- "Red flag" symptoms warrant extra attention and could indicate a more severe issue.
- Diagnostic methods for IBS include medical history evaluation, physical examination, and additional tests depending on the individual.
- Conditions that resemble or overlap with IBS include celiac disease, inflammatory bowel disease, diverticulitis, colon cancer, functional dyspepsia, lactose intolerance, small intestinal bacterial overgrowth (SIBO), sucrase-isomaltase deficiency (SID), fibromyalgia, and chronic fatigue syndrome.
- IBS also affects children and presents differently than in adults.
- Consult a healthcare professional regarding IBS symptoms if you observe warning signs or if the symptoms interfere with daily activities.

CHAPTER 5

Holistic Approach to IBS

"Health is a state of complete harmony of the body, mind, and spirit. When one is free from physical disabilities and mental distractions, the gates of the soul open." - B.K.S. Iyengar

The mind-body connection - seeing the whole person

Holistic medicine, with roots in ancient healing traditions like Ayurveda, Traditional Chinese Medicine, and indigenous practices, looks at the whole picture instead of just individual symptoms. A holistic approach considers the mind, body, and spirit working together for better health.

The mind-body connection has been around in medicine for ages. For example, Hippocrates, the ancient Greek doctor known as the father of Western medicine, was all about a holistic approach, stressing good nutrition, exercise, and emotional well-being. The ancient Greeks knew that the mind and body were linked and treated physical and mental issues as one system. Modern research keeps showing how our physical health and emotions are interconnected.

Somatization: when feelings become physical

Simply put, somatization is the phenomenon where emotional or mental stress manifests itself as physical symptoms in the body. It is worth noting that IBS can be impacted by somatization, meaning that your stress levels and emotional state can affect the severity of your IBS symptoms.

That is where holistic medicine, or "Integrated care," comes in. For IBS, it means looking at the whole person—mind, body, and spirit—instead of just the physical stuff. By tackling the emotional and mental factors that might be causing IBS through somatization, a holistic approach aims to help you manage your condition better.

A holistic plan might include stress-busting techniques like meditation, yoga, or deep-breathing exercises. By learning to handle stress and emotions better, you might see an improvement in your IBS symptoms. A holistic approach could involve talking to a therapist or counselor to dig into any emotional issues affecting your IBS.

Holistic medicine's role in IBS Management: mind, body, and spirit

Traditional IBS treatments usually focus on easing individual symptoms. Lately, though, there's been a renewed interest in holistic medicine to manage tricky, long-term conditions like IBS. For some medical issues, a holistic approach is not needed. A bacterial infection, for example, can be sorted out with antibiotics, and there is no need to bring in psychologists or dietitians. A broken bone can be handled by an orthopedic doctor who sets the bone and deals with pain management. IBS, on the other hand, is more complicated and often needs a multi-layered approach. That's because diet, stress, and emotional well-being can influence IBS symptoms.

Here are some reasons why considering the whole person is essential:

- **Mind:** The mind plays a significant role in IBS, with stress, anxiety, and depression often exacerbating symptoms. By addressing the mental aspects of IBS, individuals can better manage their stress and emotions, ultimately reducing symptom severity.

- **Body:** The physical aspect of IBS involves the gastrointestinal system and its functions. A holistic approach emphasizes the importance of a proper balance of gut bacteria, a suitable diet, and regular exercise. It encourages physical activity to improve overall health and well-being.

- **Spirit:** The spiritual aspect of a holistic approach to IBS involves finding meaning, purpose, and connection in one's life. This may include engaging in activities like meditation, yoga, or spiritual counseling to foster a sense of inner peace and balance. By nurturing the spirit, individuals may find greater resilience and ability to cope with the challenges of living with IBS.

Scientific evidence backs the holistic approach

A recent study in New York tested a treatment plan for individuals with IBS that combined diet changes and mind-body therapies in a group setting for four weeks, followed by eight weeks of phone health coaching. The study found that these individuals experienced improved symptoms compared to a control group, but overall quality of life did not differ greatly.

Holistic approaches to IBS treatment are not often studied on a large scale due to the challenges of delivering care across various specialties and settings. However, many studies support the benefits of individual therapies such as diet and stress management for IBS, suggesting that a combination of these methods may lead to even better symptom control and overall quality of life. Therefore, pursuing a holistic or integrated care approach to IBS treatment is important for optimal results.

Real-life example: Alyssa's journey to holistic healing

Alyssa, a 28-year-old woman, had been struggling with IBS for years. She was seen by a few doctors, including her primary care provider and a gastroenterologist. Her symptoms persisted and worsened over time despite trying various medications and dietary changes. Frustrated, Alyssa approached me for a 2nd opinion to discuss other options to relieve her symptoms.

By this point, she had already tried almost all the available medications. She tried a few different diets, but none worked consistently. We decided to explore a more holistic approach to her condition.

Together, we developed a comprehensive treatment plan that included dietary changes with the help of a dietician and by writing a food diary (we will discuss this later) to identify the trigger foods. We also incorporated probiotic and prebiotic supplements and stress-management techniques like yoga and meditation. Alyssa also started attending weekly therapy sessions to address her anxiety, which she discovered exacerbated her IBS symptoms.

Over time, Alyssa's symptoms began to improve. As she learned to manage her stress and anxiety, her IBS symptoms became more manageable. This holistic approach helped her physical symptoms and overall mental and emotional well-being.

What's involved in a holistic approach to IBS?

A holistic IBS approach means more than just seeing a gastroenterologist. A team of healthcare professionals can help you handle IBS way better. Let's check out the roles of different experts in this approach.

Dietician: They can help you figure out and cut trigger foods from your diet while ensuring you still eat healthy and manage your IBS symptoms.

Gastrointestinal psychologist: They understand the gut-brain connection and can help you find ways to deal with stress and anxiety, which can worsen IBS symptoms.

Counselor: They offer emotional support and help you tackle the challenges of living with IBS. Plus, they help you learn to communicate better, especially when discussing your condition with family or co-workers.

Hypnotherapist: Hypnotherapy can help you relax and stress less, which can help with IBS symptoms. Some people with IBS find relief through hypnotherapy because it helps them handle pain and discomfort more effectively.

Cognitive-behavioral therapy (CBT) therapist: CBT can help you change negative thoughts and behaviors that might worsen your IBS. A CBT therapist can teach you techniques to manage stress and anxiety better, leading to improved symptom control.

Making holistic medicine easy and approachable

Holistic medicine might seem intimidating, especially if you are used to conventional treatments. But going holistic for IBS doesn't have to be complicated. It can be as simple as changing your diet gradually, adding stress management techniques to your daily routine, and getting psychological support when needed.

A key part of making holistic medicine more approachable is ensuring patients and healthcare providers know the benefits. By giving clear, easy-to-understand information about the different parts of a holistic treatment plan, patients can feel in control of their health and make smart choices about their care.

Managing IBS through a holistic approach or integrated care is a promising and well-supported method to address this complex condition. By looking at the whole person – mind, body, and spirit – and understanding the connections between the gut, brain, and emotions, people with IBS can see significant improvements in their symptoms and overall life quality.

As research continues and more people become aware of holistic medicine's benefits, this approach will become a crucial tool against IBS and other long-term conditions. The following chapters will dive into each component of holistic approach, including diet, psychological therapies, and complementary and alternative meds. We will also discuss over the counter and prescription medications for IBS management.

CHAPTER 6

Dietary changes for IBS

"The food you eat can either be the safest and most powerful form of medicine or the slowest form of poison." - Ann Wigmore

The kitchen fix: discover health solutions beyond your medicine cabinet

As a doctor trained in modern medicine, I have spent years prescribing medications for various health issues. But after three decades of research and listening to my patients, I have realized that many cures aren't in the medicine cabinet but in our pantry and fridge. There are studies showing how changes in diet and lifestyle can prevent or treat various health issues. Unfortunately, many individuals do not adopt healthier eating habits due to obstacles such as expense, effort, or lack of knowledge.

For people with IBS food sensitivities can be especially challenging. Research indicates that up to half of IBS patients react poorly to certain foods. Every meal feels like a gamble for them: "will it cause a flare-up or go down smoothly?"

Many people try to handle their symptoms by identifying triggers through trial and error. In one survey, over half of IBS patients had cut out specific foods, and 25% had tried going gluten-free.

Patients often ask me if they should get food allergy testing since they react to many foods. But testing for food allergies in IBS patients isn't reliable, as these tests often give false results. Adults usually don't develop many food allergies all of a sudden, and IBS patients aren't more likely to have them. In addition, allergy tests like serum IgE levels and skin prick tests are not accurate for food sensitivities. So, testing IBS patients for food allergies is not efficient or cost-effective.

The low-FODMAP diet

The Low-FODMAP diet was first introduced in 2005 by Australian researchers at Monash University. FODMAP stands for Fermentable Oligosaccharides, Disaccharides, Monosaccharides, and Polyols. These are short-chain carbohydrates that are not easily absorbed by the small intestine. When these carbs are fermented by bacteria in the large intestine, it can cause bloating, gas, and abdominal pain for people who have IBS.

High-FODMAP foods include wheat, onions, garlic, dairy, legumes, and certain fruits and vegetables. This diet has become popular as a potential solution for digestive issues like IBS. Even though it can be challenging to follow, it has the most robust scientific evidence supporting its effectiveness.

Scientific evidence

Many studies have looked at the Low-FODMAP diet's effectiveness in managing IBS symptoms, with some saying up to 75% of people see improvements. A thorough review and analysis of multiple randomized controlled trials showed the diet significantly reduced IBS symptoms like bloating, abdominal pain, and diarrhea.

How to follow low-FODMAP diet plan:

- Restrict high-FODMAP foods (lasting 4-6 weeks)
- Reintroduce FODMAP foods
- Personalize based on reintroduction results (using a food diary to track reactions to specific foods and create a tailored meal plan)

Pros and cons of the low-FODMAP Diet:

Pros:

o Safe and effective for managing IBS symptoms
o Reduces symptoms like bloating, gas, and abdominal pain
o May improve overall gut health and quality of life
o All-natural approach
o Easy to follow with a dietitian or nutritionist's guidance

Cons:

o Difficult to maintain, particularly for food lovers or frequent restaurant-goers
o Restricts many nutrient-rich foods, potentially leading to poor nutrient intake and long-term risk of inadequate calcium and vitamin D
o Alters gut bacteria, potentially causing damage to the long-term health of the gut
o May cause food anxiety or stress
o Eliminating certain foods can lead to social stress or isolation

Tips for following the low-FODMAP diet:

- Work with a registered dietitian to ensure proper execution and nutrient intake
- Keep a food diary to track symptoms and identify trigger foods
- Read food labels carefully to avoid high-FODMAP ingredients
- Try low-FODMAP alternatives to high-FODMAP foods
- Gradually reintroduce high-FODMAP foods to pinpoint trigger foods
- You can find more information about the Monash University Low FODMAP Diet on their official website:
  https://www.monashfodmap.com/
- Monash University's Low-FODMAP diet app offers a comprehensive list of high and low-FODMAP foods, recipes, and meal plans for easier adherence.

Links to download the app:

For iOS devices (iPhone and iPad): https://apps.apple.com/us/app/monash-university-fodmap-diet/id586149216

For Android devices: https://play.google.com/store/apps/details?id=com.monashuniversity.fodmap&hl=en_US&gl=US

Examples of high-FODMAP diets and their low-FODMAP diet alternatives

Food Type	High-FODMAP Foods	Low-FODMAP Alternatives
Fruits	Apples, pears, peaches, Mangoes, cherries, plums	Strawberries, grapes, oranges, blueberries, raspberries, bananas (unripe)
Vegetables	Onions, garlic, cabbage, asparagus, cauliflower	Bell peppers, carrots, cucumber, green beans, zucchini, spinach
Meats	Sausages, marinated meats, processed deli meats	Plain chicken, beef, pork, fresh fish, eggs, tofu
Bread	Wheat bread, rye bread	Gluten-free bread, rice cakes
Grains	Barley, couscous, wheat	Corn, rice, quinoa
Pasta	Wheat pasta	Gluten-free pasta, rice noodles
Dairy	Cow's milk, soft cheese, yogurt, ice cream	Lactose-free milk, hard cheese, almond milk, lactose-free yogurt
Nuts & Seeds	Cashews, pistachios	Almonds, walnuts, pumpkin seeds
Sweeteners	Honey, high fructose corn syrup, agave syrup, xylitol	Maple syrup, table sugar, stevia, erythritol

Keep in mind that FODMAP tolerance is different for everyone. Work with a dietitian to determine which foods are best for you.

To sum up, the Low-FODMAP diet can help with IBS symptoms, but it can be risky if followed for too long. Don't stick to the diet for a long time without professional supervision. Try to bring back high-FODMAP foods now and then to avoid an overly strict diet.

Lactose-free diet

Lactose intolerance occurs when your body lacks the lactase enzyme to break down lactose in the gut, leading to symptoms such as gas, bloating, and diarrhea. Interestingly, these symptoms resemble those of IBS, so it is crucial to investigate how the two conditions are related. Lactose intolerance is widespread, affecting up to 75% of the global population.

I often recommend a lactose-free diet as the initial step for newly diagnosed IBS patients, particularly those of African American, Hispanic, Native American, or Mediterranean (Arab, Jewish, Greek, and Italian) descent, who are more likely to be lactose intolerant. It is conceivable that some of these individuals' IBS symptoms may be due to lactose intolerance. Furthermore, a lactose-free diet is generally easy to follow because many lactose-free options are available. This way, patients can quickly determine if it is effective, and if not, they can try another diet or treatment. However, keep in mind that there isn't enough scientific evidence to suggest that a low-lactose or lactose-free diet is suitable for everyone with IBS.

Tips for a successful lactose-free diet

Read food labels carefully: Look for hidden lactose in prepared foods, including those with evaporated or condensed milk and buttermilk.

Choose lactose-free or lactose-reduced dairy products: Plenty of dairy alternatives are easy to find in most supermarkets, making a lactose-free diet more manageable.

Include other calcium and vitamin D sources in your diet: This helps ensure you get the nutrients you need even if you are not eating lactose.

Gradually reduce lactose: Don't make sudden diet changes; keep track of symptom relief as you lower your lactose intake.

Talk to the professionals: Before trying a lactose-free diet for IBS, it is crucial to chat with a healthcare professional or registered dietitian. They can advise you on keeping a balanced diet, ensuring you get the nutrients you need, sticking to a lactose-free diet, and suggesting other sources of calcium and nutrients. Following their guidance, you can make sure your lactose-free diet is healthy and meets your nutritional needs.

Gluten-free diet

A gluten-free diet means avoiding gluten, a protein found in certain foods. This diet is popular, and many people use it to deal with IBS.

Why go gluten-free for IBS?

A gluten-free diet can help some patients with IBS by reducing or eliminating their exposure to gluten, a protein found in wheat, barley, and rye. This sensitivity is different from celiac disease, which is an autoimmune disorder where the ingestion of gluten leads to damage in the small intestine. For certain individuals, gluten can trigger IBS symptoms, even if they do not have celiac disease.

The exact mechanism through which gluten affects IBS is not fully understood, but it is believed to involve several factors:

1. **Gluten sensitivity:** Some individuals with IBS may have non-celiac gluten sensitivity (NCGS) or a wheat allergy, a condition where they experience symptoms similar to those of celiac disease but without the autoimmune response that damages the small intestine. In such cases, following a gluten-free diet can alleviate IBS symptoms.

2. **FODMAPs:** Gluten-containing grains, such as wheat, barley, and rye, are also high in FODMAPs. Patients who follow a gluten-free diet may unknowingly decrease their consumption of FODMAPs, which could lead to an improvement in their symptoms.

3. **Gut inflammation:** Gluten may contribute to low-grade inflammation in the gut, exacerbating IBS symptoms in some individuals. Removing gluten from the diet can help reduce this inflammation and alleviate IBS symptoms.

Scientific evidence

Studies show that going gluten-free can help certain people with IBS. A small 2013 study with 45 patients found that a gluten-free diet improved overall symptoms in people with IBS-D (IBS with diarrhea) compared to a control diet. Another study showed that a gluten-free diet improved the quality of life and gut symptoms in people with IBS.

Pros and cons of a gluten-free diet for IBS:

Going gluten-free for IBS can help some patients with NCGS and may help reduce inflammation in the gut. But cutting out wheat, barley, and rye can lead to nutrient deficiencies. Gluten-free products can also be more expensive and harder to find than stuff with gluten.

Tips for a gluten-free diet for IBS:

- Read food labels carefully to make sure products are gluten-free
- Stick to naturally gluten-free foods like fruits, veggies, lean proteins, and gluten-free grains like quinoa and rice
- Avoid processed gluten-free foods that can be high in calories and low in nutrients

- Talk to a registered dietitian to make sure you are getting all the nutrients you need

High-fiber diet

A high-fiber diet, especially with lots of soluble fiber, can be great for people with IBS.

Why go with high-fiber diet?

Fiber is crucial for maintaining good digestive health, but it can be troublesome for those with IBS if consumed in excessive amounts. As a carbohydrate that our bodies cannot break down, fiber passes through our system largely unaltered, adding bulk to our stool and promoting regular bowel movements.

Fiber is found in plant-based foods like fruits, veggies, nuts, whole grains, and seeds, and comes in two forms- soluble and insoluble. Soluble fiber, which dissolves in water, forms a gel-like substance that helps alleviate IBS symptoms by regulating bowel movements, improving stool consistency, and reducing gas and bloating. On the other hand, for those with IBS, too much insoluble fiber can cause increased gas, bloating, and discomfort. Foods like wheat bran, whole grains, and some veggies have insoluble fiber.

Here are some good sources of soluble fiber:

- **Oats and oat bran:** Oats are a rich source of soluble fiber, particularly a type called beta-glucan. Oat bran is the outer layer of the oat grain and is especially high in soluble fiber.
- **Legumes:** Beans, peas, and lentils are all excellent sources of soluble fiber, as well as protein and various micronutrients.

- **Fruits:** Apples, pears, oranges, and bananas are all good sources of soluble fiber. The fiber is found primarily in the fruit's skin and flesh.
- **Vegetables:** Some vegetables, such as carrots, Brussels sprouts, and sweet potatoes, contain significant amounts of soluble fiber.
- **Psyllium husk:** Derived from the seeds of the Plantago ovata plant, psyllium husk is a popular supplement known for its high soluble fiber content.
- **Flaxseeds and chia seeds:** These seeds are not only rich in soluble fiber, but they also provide healthy fats and various essential nutrients.
- **Barley:** This grain is a good source of soluble fiber and can be used in various dishes, such as soups, stews, and salads.
- **Nuts:** Almonds, walnuts, and peanuts are examples of nuts that contain a moderate amount of soluble fiber.

Scientific evidence

Studies have shown that eating more fiber can help with IBS symptoms. In a 2014 study from the Netherlands, researchers found that the soluble fiber supplement psyllium significantly improved IBS symptoms compared to a placebo. After three months of treatment, symptom severity in the psyllium group dropped by 90 points, compared with 49 points in the placebo group. Another study, which compiled 12 different studies, showed that Ispaghula (another name for psyllium) improved IBS symptoms compared to a placebo.

How does the high-fiber diet help IBS?

A high-fiber diet not only adds bulk to your stool, helping it move through your digestive system more efficiently but also fosters the growth of beneficial bacteria in your gut, improving digestion and reducing inflammation.

Benefits of a high-fiber diet

- Improved bowel regularity
- Reduced constipation
- Decreased abdominal pain and bloating
- Enhanced overall bowel function
- Lower risk of colon cancer
- Regulation of blood sugar and cholesterol

Tips for a high-fiber diet

If you are considering a high-fiber diet for IBS, follow these tips:

- Focus on soluble fiber and avoid insoluble fiber
- Watch out for worsening of bloating symptoms if you consume excessive fiber
- Add fiber to your diet gradually
- Consume high-fiber foods like fruits, vegetables, whole grains, nuts, and seeds
- Drink lots of water to help your body adjust to more fiber
- Collaborate with a registered dietitian to create a personalized high-fiber meal plan

Adults should aim for 25-35 grams of fiber per day, although this might vary depending on individual needs and health conditions.

Foods high in soluble fiber

Food	Serving Size	Fiber Content
Psyllium husk	1 tablespoon	5 grams
Chia seeds	1 ounce	10 grams
Flaxseeds	1 tablespoon	3 grams
Barley	1 cup	6 grams
Lentils	1/2 cup	8 grams
Peas	1/2 cup	4 grams
Sweet potato	1 medium	4 grams
Brussels sprouts	1 cup	4 grams
Broccoli	1 cup	2.6 grams
Chickpeas	1/2 cup	6 grams
Baked beans, canned, no salt added	1 cup	14 grams
Carrots	1 medium	2 grams
Apples	1 medium	4 grams
Berries	1 cup	Strawberries (2gm), Blueberries (4gm), Raspberries (8 gm)
Oranges	1 medium	3 grams

Starch and sucrose-reduced diet

Many individuals with IBS have unhealthy eating habits, consuming cereals, sweets, and soft drinks at random times while not consuming enough vegetables, fruits, and fish. Research has shown a correlation between soft drink consumption and digestive issues. Some individuals with IBS may experience symptoms due to their poor diet rather than a bowel problem.

Dietary sugars can cause inflammation and gut leakiness, which are associated with IBS. These sugars can ferment in the gut, leading to gas, bloating, cramping, and diarrhea. Reducing the intake of sugars such as sucrose (table sugar), fructose, and starches found in bread, pasta, and potatoes may be beneficial for individuals with IBS.

Scientific evidence

Research has indicated that reducing starch and sugar intake may be effective in managing IBS symptoms. In a 2019 study, a four-week reduction in these dietary components (known as a Starch and Sucrose reduced Diet, or SSD) led to symptom reduction in 74% of patients, as well as improvements in additional symptoms such as belching, fatigue, and joint pain. This resulted in an overall enhancement of psychological well-being.

Potential benefits and risks of cutting down sugars and starches

Eating less sucrose and starch might help improve digestion, reduce bloating, and decrease diarrhea episodes for people with IBS. It could also make life better overall for those suffering from IBS.

One risk of eating less sugar and starch is that you might not get enough essential nutrients like fiber, vitamins, and minerals. To avoid nutrient deficiencies, make sure your diet is balanced and has foods from all food groups.

Tips for cutting down sugars and starches

- Carefully read food labels to identify sources of sucrose and starch.
- Cut down or avoid high-sucrose and high-starch foods like candy, cakes, bread, pasta, and potatoes.

- Swap high-sucrose and high-starch foods for low-sucrose and low-starch alternatives, like fresh fruits and vegetables, lean protein, and whole grains such as quinoa and brown rice.
- Work with a registered dietitian to create a balanced, healthy meal plan that meets your nutrient needs while avoiding trigger foods.

Foods to eat:

- **Protein sources:** Lean meats, poultry, fish, eggs, tofu, and tempeh.
- **Fruits:** Choose low-sugar fruits such as berries, kiwi, and citrus fruits. Consume them in moderation.
- **Low-starch vegetables:** Leafy greens, broccoli, cauliflower, green beans, bell peppers, zucchini, cucumber, and tomatoes.
- **Nuts and seeds:** Almonds, walnuts, chia seeds, flaxseeds, and sunflower seeds.
- **Dairy or dairy alternatives:** Unsweetened yogurt, cheese, and milk or unsweetened plant-based milk alternatives like almond milk, coconut milk, or soy milk.
- **Fats and oils:** Use healthy oils like olive, avocado, and coconut oil for cooking and dressing.
- **Beverages:** Drink water, herbal teas, and black coffee without added sugars.
- **Sweeteners:** If needed, use small amounts of natural sugar substitutes, such as stevia or erythritol.

Foods to avoid or limit:

- **Sugary foods and beverages:** Avoid soft drinks, fruit juices, candies, chocolates, pastries, and desserts high in sugar.

- **High-starch vegetables:** Potatoes, sweet potatoes, yams, corn, and peas.
- **High-starch fruits:** Bananas, grapes, and pineapples.
- **Grains:** Reduce or avoid the consumption of refined grains, like white rice, white bread, and pasta. Opt for smaller portions of whole grains, such as quinoa, brown rice, and whole wheat pasta, if you include them.
- **Legumes:** Beans and lentils can be high in starch, so limit their intake or choose alternatives like chickpeas

The Elimination Diet: be a food detective to find your triggers

What is the elimination diet?

If you're not sure which diet to adhere to or if you think some foods may be exacerbating your IBS symptoms, the elimination diet can help you identify the culprits. It is a temporary process wherein you remove particular foods from your meals and monitor if your symptoms get better. You can then gradually reintroduce these foods to determine if they cause any symptoms to resurface. This technique helps you pinpoint your individual IBS triggers.

Scientific evidence

A Swedish study found that 84% of participants had symptoms related to at least one food item. Common culprits were fatty foods, dairy, beans/lentils, apples, flour, and plums. Some people also had issues with foods high in biogenic amines or histamine-releasing foods.

How does the elimination diet work?

Start by cutting out possible trigger foods for about 2-4 weeks. Usual suspects include:

- Dairy products
- Gluten-containing foods
- FODMAPs
- Caffeine
- Alcohol
- Fried or greasy foods
- Spicy foods
- Chocolate
- Carbonated drinks
- Wheat
- Beans and legumes
- Foods high in biogenic amines or histamine-releasing foods (fermented foods, aged cheeses, processed meats, canned fish, dried fruits like figs, raisins, apricots, and prunes or even storing leftovers in the refrigerator for too long might elevate histamine levels).

It is important to note that not all these foods will cause problems for everyone with IBS. While it can be challenging to identify the problematic foods, keeping a food diary can help you pinpoint your specific triggers. After the elimination phase, gradually reintroduce foods one by one to determine if they cause any issues.

Tips for the elimination diet

- Work with a registered dietitian for a personalized plan.
- Keep a food diary to track symptoms and potential triggers.
- Be patient and committed—it takes time to identify triggers and see improvements.
- Get creative with ingredients and cooking methods to enjoy your meals.

- Reintroduce foods slowly and one at a time to accurately identify triggers.
- Monitor symptoms and note which foods cause them.

Fermented foods and probiotic power

Fermented foods like yogurt, kefir, kombucha, sauerkraut, kimchi, tempeh, and miso are full of live microorganisms, some are similar to strains found in probiotics. While there are not many clinical studies on fermented foods, available evidence suggests that they offer health benefits beyond their original food sources.

Scientific evidence

Studies show probiotics can ease IBS symptoms like bloating, gas, and constipation. A 2015 review of 35 studies found that probiotics significantly reduced IBS symptoms, including bloating and flatulence. Another study showed that a probiotic supplement lessened abdominal pain and improved bowel movements in people with IBS.

There is some evidence that kefir may help some digestive symptoms, but no clinical trials have been done to prove its effectiveness. Kombucha is a fermented tea drink that has become popular for its potential health benefits, including improving gut health. It is made by fermenting sweetened tea with a symbiotic culture of bacteria and yeast (SCOBY). During fermentation, the SCOBY consumes sugar, producing a slightly fizzy and tangy drink rich in probiotics, organic acids, and antioxidants.

The probiotics in kombucha may help alleviate IBS symptoms by improving gut flora balance and promoting a healthy digestive system. However, scientific research on the specific effects of kombucha on IBS is limited. Most evidence supporting fermented foods' benefits on IBS comes from studies on other probiotic-rich foods or supplements.

Fermented food ideas

- **Yogurt:** Go for plain yogurt with live active cultures, avoiding added sugars or artificial sweeteners. Greek yogurt is also a good choice because it is strained and typically has higher protein content.
- **Kefir:** A fermented milk drink packed with various beneficial bacteria and yeasts.
- **Kimchi:** A traditional spicy and tangy Korean dish made from fermented veggies, usually cabbage.
- **Sauerkraut:** A fermented vegetable dish typically made from cabbage. It has a sour taste and can be used as a topping for salads or sandwiches.
- **Kombucha:** A fermented tea often flavored with fruit juice, containing various beneficial bacteria and yeasts.

If you plan to try fermented foods, watch for side effects, as not everyone tolerates them.

- **Digestive issues:** Some people might experience gas, bloating, or stomach cramps when they first consume fermented foods. This is usually temporary and might subside once the body adjusts to the new food source.
- **Allergic reactions:** In rare cases, people might be allergic to certain ingredients in fermented foods, which could lead to an allergic reaction.
- **High sodium content:** Some fermented foods, like pickles and sauerkraut, can have a high sodium content. This can be a con-

cern for people who need to watch their salt intake due to high blood pressure or other health issues.

- **Histamine intolerance:** Fermented foods can contain high levels of histamine that can cause problems for people who are sensitive to histamine or have histamine intolerance.
- **Contamination risk:** Homemade fermented foods might have a higher risk of contamination if proper hygiene and food safety practices are not followed. This could lead to foodborne illnesses.

Precautions to take when consuming fermented foods

- **Start slow:** Introduce fermented foods into your diet gradually, allowing your body to adjust to the new food source.
- **Pay attention to portion sizes:** Consume moderate portions of fermented foods, as overconsumption could cause digestive issues.
- **Choose low-sodium options:** If you are concerned about salt intake, opt for low-sodium varieties of fermented foods, or make your own at home using less salt.
- **Be cautious with histamine:** If you have histamine intolerance or sensitivity, avoid, or limit your consumption of high-histamine fermented foods (like aged cheeses, vinegar-containing foods, etc.).
- **Practice good hygiene and food safety:** When making fermented foods at home, follow proper food safety guidelines to minimize the risk of contamination.

Fixing a leaky gut: easy ways to boost gut health

- Eat a balanced diet with fiber, whole grains, fruits, and veggies. This helps good gut bacteria thrive, keeping your intestinal barrier strong. Avoid processed and inflammatory foods like sugary snacks, white bread, fried goodies, and red meat.
- Stress less. Long-term stress can harm your intestinal barrier, increasing the risk of a leaky gut. Keep stress in check with exercise, mindfulness techniques, or chatting with someone you trust to keep your gut feeling great.
- Watch out for certain medications and chemicals. Avoiding nonsteroidal anti-inflammatory drugs (NSAIDs) and antibiotics can help maintain a healthy intestinal barrier.
- Think about glutamine supplements. This amino acid can fix the gut lining and tighten up the junctions. A small study in 2019 found that taking 5 grams of glutamine three times a day made a big difference for patients with PI-IBS.

Tackling the Candida: the anti-Candida diet

The anti-Candida diet aims to restrict the growth of Candida in your gut by eliminating foods that promote its growth and introducing foods that restore balance. This involves avoiding high-sugar foods, refined carbs, alcohol, and moldy foods that can increase Candida growth. Instead, focus on nutrient-dense, anti-inflammatory foods like vegetables, healthy fats, lean proteins, and low-glycemic fruits.

Scientific evidence

The scientific evidence for the effectiveness of the anti-Candida diet is mixed. The link between gastrointestinal Candida colonization and IBS is still being studied. Some research suggests a correlation, while other studies do not find a significant connection. Further research is necessary to understand the role of Candida overgrowth in IBS. However, certain aspects of the diet, such as consuming fiber-rich fruits and vegetables, can be beneficial for gut health by promoting a healthy gut microbiome and reducing inflammation.

Top tips for the anti-Candida diet

Principle	Tips	Suggested Recipes
1. Skip sugar & artificial sweeteners	Avoid sugar, honey, maple syrup, and agave nectar. Choose stevia or xylitol moderately.	Stevia smoothies, xylitol desserts
2. Go low carb	Pick leafy greens, broccoli, cauliflower, and zucchini. No bread, pasta, or potatoes.	Cauliflower stir-fry, zucchini noodles with pesto
3. Lean protein only	Opt for chicken, fish, or tofu. Steer clear of bacon and sausage.	Grilled chicken & roasted veggies, baked salmon & quinoa
4. Healthy fats	Add avocado, nuts, and seeds. Avoid trans fats and vegetable oils.	Avocado toast & almond butter, mixed nut trail mix
5. Probiotics, please	Eat yogurt, kefir, sauerkraut. Skip sugary yogurts.	Plain Greek yogurt & berries, sauerkraut on salad
6. Ditch dairy	Avoid milk and cheese. Choose almond milk and cashew cheese.	Almond milk smoothies, cashew cheese & veggie sandwich

7. Cut caffeine & alcohol	Limit coffee and alcohol. Drink herbal teas and sparkling water.	Chamomile tea, sparkling water & lemon
8. Anti-fungal foods	Eat garlic, coconut oil, and ginger to fight Candida.	Garlic shrimp stir-fry, coconut oil roasted veggies
9. Hydrate	Drink water to flush toxins and support detox.	Lemon water, herbal tea
10. Mindful eating	Listen to hunger and fullness cues. No mindless snacking.	Roasted almonds, veggies & hummus

Which diet should I try for my IBS?

Are you confused about which diet to follow for IBS? Unfortunately, there is no one-size-fits-all solution. Low-FODMAP diet is the most researched and proven diet although maintaining it can be challenging.

As a starting point, you could try a lactose-free diet for two weeks. If that doesn't help, you could try a gluten-free or low-FODMAP diet, depending on your preferences. Generally, a gluten-free diet is easier to follow and should be tried for four weeks. If that doesn't work, the next option is a low-FODMAP diet. If you find the low-FODMAP diet too challenging or ineffective, there are other diets to consider, such as high-fiber, SSD, elimination, anti-candida, or leaky gut diets. It is important to remember that everyone's experience with IBS is unique, so it may take some trial and error to find the best diet for you.

NICE guidelines for IBS

The National Institute for Health and Care Excellence (NICE) is a UK-based organization that provides evidence-based guidelines for various health conditions, including IBS.

What are the NICE IBS diet guidelines?

The NICE IBS diet guidelines aim to help people with IBS manage their symptoms by making simple changes to their eating habits. The guidelines suggest general dietary advice as well as specific recommendations tailored to an individual's symptoms.

What to Eat and What to Avoid:

1. **Eat regular meals:** Have meals at regular intervals and avoid skipping meals or eating large meals. This helps your gut maintain a consistent routine, which may reduce IBS symptoms.

2. **Limit high-fat foods:** Cut down on fatty and fried foods, as they can contribute to IBS symptoms like bloating and diarrhea.

3. **Be mindful of fiber:** If you suffer from constipation, gradually increase your fiber intake by including more whole grains, fruits, and vegetables in your diet. However, if you have diarrhea, reduce your intake of high-fiber foods.

4. **Stay hydrated:** Drink plenty of water throughout the day, aiming for at least 8 cups (2 liters) of fluid daily.

5. **Limit caffeine:** Cut back on caffeine from coffee, tea, and energy drinks, as it can trigger IBS symptoms.

6. **Avoid gas-producing foods:** Some people with IBS may experience worsening symptoms with gas-producing foods like beans, lentils, onions, and cabbage. Monitor your symptoms and adjust your diet accordingly.

7. **Be cautious with lactose:** If you suspect lactose intolerance, try reducing or eliminating dairy products from your diet to see if your symptoms improve.
8. **Watch out for artificial sweeteners:** Some sugar-free products contain sweeteners like sorbitol and mannitol, which can worsen IBS symptoms.
9. **Consider a low-FODMAP diet.**

Nutrition and meal planning for IBS

Food and symptom diary

Keeping a food and symptom diary can help you identify IBS triggers and track how factors like stress or sleep affect your condition. Use this information to make adjustments and discuss your findings with your healthcare provider.

- **Keep a food diary:** Your key to unlocking IBS relief
- **Pick your diary style:** Choose a method that is easy for you, like a notebook, digital document, or app. Make sure you can access and update it daily.
- **Write down everything you eat:** For every entry, note the date, time, food, portion size, and symptoms. Be thorough, listing ingredients, condiments, and drinks. Don't forget the emotional or physical factors that could affect your IBS, like stress, sleep, or exercise.
- **Rate your discomfort:** After each meal, score your symptoms (abdominal pain, bloating, gas, diarrhea, or constipation) from 1 to 10.
- **Spot the triggers:** Look for patterns in your diary after a few weeks. Identify foods, ingredients, emotions, stress, or sleep

issues that worsen your IBS. Share your findings with your healthcare provider for more guidance.

- **Tweak your diet:** Armed with your trigger list, adjust your diet to cut out or minimize those foods. Reintroduce the foods that you find that you are tolerating well so that you will have more food choices.

- Links to sample tables in PDF form that can be printed and used for keeping a food diary:

https://irritablebowelsyndrome.net/wp-content/uploads/2022/06/IBS-Food-Journal-Downloadable-PDF-2022.pdf?utm_source=IBSFJ

https://www.ibsdiets.org/wp-content/uploads/2015/05/fodmap-food-diary.pdf

Sample table for a food diary:

Date	Time	Meal/ Snack	Abdominal Pain (1-10)	Bloating (1-10)	Gas (1-10)	Diarrhea (1-10)	Constipation (1-10)	Notes (foods, stress, activity)
01/01/2022	8AM	Breakfast	2	3	2	1		Oatmeal, almond milk, banana
01/01/2022	12 PM	Lunch	5	6		2		Grilled chicken, salad, vinaigrette dressing
01/01/2022	3 PM	Snack	2	2	2			Carrots, hummus
01/01/2022	7 PM	Dinner	7	8	4	3		Spaghetti with tomato sauce, garlic bread

Note: The "Notes" column can record additional information about the meal or snack, such as specific foods, stress levels, or physical activity.

You can use several digital apps to track the symptoms and their link to IBS symptoms. Some examples-

1. mySymptoms food diary & symptom tracker

   iOS: https://apps.apple.com/us/app/mysymptoms-food-diary

   Android: https://play.google.com/store/apps/mysymptoms

2. Cara Care: IBS tracker & gut health

   iOS: https://apps.apple.com/us/app/cara-care-ibs-tracker

   Android: https://play.google.com/store/CaraCare

3. Bowelle:

   iOS: https://apps.apple.com/us/app/bowelle-the-ibs-tracker

Eating out and social events

Choosing restaurants and menus:

- **Do some homework:** Find IBS-friendly restaurants or places catering to dietary restrictions.
- **Peek at the menu:** Check menus in advance to find suitable dishes.
- **Make a call:** Discuss your needs and ask about menu adjustments with the restaurant.

Tackling buffets and potlucks:

- **Survey the scene:** Spot IBS-friendly dishes among the options.
- **Avoid trouble:** Skip fried, spicy, or trigger foods.
- **Keep it simple:** Fill your plate with basic foods and small portions to minimize symptoms.

Alcohol and IBS:

- **Tread carefully:** Choose low-alcohol options like light beer or wine and drink moderately.

- **Pair wisely:** Always eat food with alcohol and stay hydrated.
- **Mind the mixers:** Watch out for sugar or triggers in cocktail mixers.

Building a support network:

- **Share your story:** Tell friends and family about your IBS journey so that they can support you at social events.

Recipe adaptation

- **Swap the bad:** Replace trigger ingredients with gut-friendly alternatives.
- **Flavor it up:** Experiment with herbs and spices for taste.
- **Dairy swaps:** Use lactose-free or plant-based alternatives when needed.
- **Batch cooking and freezing.**
- **Cook big:** Prepare large quantities of IBS-friendly meals and freeze single servings.
- **Stock up:** Have a meal ready when busy or tired with freezer-friendly meals like soups, stews, casseroles, and cooked grains.

Meal planning resources:

- **Get inspired:** Use IBS-friendly cookbooks, blogs, and forums for meal ideas and tips.
- **Connect with others:** Share recipes and support with fellow IBS sufferers.
- **Balancing Nutrition and Variety.**
- **Plan wisely:** IBS-friendly meals include protein, healthy fats, and complex carbs.

- **Keep it fresh:** Try new foods and ingredients to maintain variety.
- **Get essential nutrients:** Incorporate gut-friendly fruits, veggies, and whole grains for vitamins and minerals.

Helpful IBS resources:

- International Foundation for Gastrointestinal Disorders (IFFGD): https://www.iffgd.org/
- Monash University Low-FODMAP Diet: https://www.monash-fodmap.com/
- Academy of Nutrition and Dietetics: https://www.eatright.org/
- National Institute of Diabetes and Digestive and Kidney Diseases (NIDDK): https://www.niddk.nih.gov/health-information/digestive-diseases/irritable-bowel-syndrome/treatment
- American College of Gastroenterology (ACG): https://gi.org/

CHAPTER 7

Mind-body Therapy Techniques for IBS

"The mind is everything; what you think, you become." – Buddha

A happy brain is equal to a happy gut

The connection between the mind and body is especially significant when it comes to IBS. As discussed in previous chapters, when you have IBS, your brain and gut are not working well together as they should. For instance, feelings of stress or anxiety can trigger symptoms such as stomach cramps, diarrhea, or constipation. Conversely, digestive issues can impact one's mood and cause feelings of worry or distress. Therefore, it is crucial to focus on both the physical and mental aspects of IBS management. This can be achieved by maintaining a healthy diet that is gentle on your digestive system, exercising regularly, and getting sufficient sleep. Additionally, relaxation techniques such as deep breathing, yoga, or meditation can help you calm your mind and alleviate stress.

Taming your tummy: gut-directed psychotherapies

Gut-directed psychotherapies (GDPs) may include many forms of therapy. We will discuss the three most common forms of GDPs-

1. Cognitive-behavioral therapy (CBT)
2. Gut-directed hypnotherapy

3. Mindfulness-based stress reduction

Cognitive-behavioral therapy (CBT)

CBT is a therapeutic approach that addresses negative thinking patterns and behaviors associated with mental health challenges such as anxiety and depression. It is based on the understanding that thoughts, emotions, and actions are interconnected and mutually influence each other.

CBT aims to help people spot and change unhelpful thoughts leading to negative emotions and behavior. For instance, anxiety can stem from thoughts like "I'm not good enough" or "I will fail," causing insecurity and avoidance behaviors.

With weekly one-on-one sessions, a therapist helps you pinpoint negative thoughts and behaviors. Together, you will create positive, realistic ways of thinking and learn coping strategies. CBT can effectively address depression, anxiety disorders, eating disorders, and obsessive-compulsive disorder.

CBT for IBS

CBT can be invaluable for IBS in managing symptoms and enhancing the quality of life. Mental health professionals teach techniques like understanding the gut-brain connection, relaxation and stress management, and challenging negative IBS-related thoughts.

What to expect from CBT for IBS

Generally, CBT for IBS covers the following:

*   *Cognitive restructuring:* Identify and replace negative IBS-related thoughts with helpful, realistic ones.

- *Relaxation training*: Learn techniques like deep breathing and progressive muscle relaxation to reduce stress and anxiety.
- *Behavioral strategies*: Make changes to behaviors affecting IBS symptoms, like avoiding trigger foods or increasing physical activity.
- *Mindfulness*: Practice "being present" and observing thoughts and emotions without judgment to reduce stress and enhance well-being.

CBT and its many forms

CBT comes in various formats:

1. In-person therapy
2. Self-administered
3. Telephone-based therapy
4. Online therapy

Your choice depends upon factors like accessibility, preference, and symptom severity.

In-person CBT

In-person CBT involves weekly meetings with a trained therapist to discuss thoughts and feelings related to IBS. They teach techniques to change negative thinking patterns and develop healthier coping methods. In-person CBT offers a personalized experience, but other forms can be effective and more convenient for some people.

Self-administered

Self-administered CBT involves working through materials alone, without a therapist. Minimal contact CBT (MC-CBT) is similar but includes some therapist guidance in person, by phone, or online. MC-CBT uses self-help materials like worksheets, exercises, and recordings to teach symptom management skills. The therapist helps set goals, monitor progress, and provide feedback.

Telephone-based CBT

This format of CBT conducted over the phone suits people who have difficulty accessing in-person therapy or prefer phone communication. Telephone-based CBT effectively treats mental health conditions like depression, anxiety, and PTSD and might work for IBS too.

Online CBT

CBT via the internet delivers therapy sessions and materials through email, chat, or video conferencing. It has proven effective for various mental health conditions and might also help IBS sufferers.

Complementary therapies with CBT

Other techniques may be used in addition to CBT based on individual profiles and therapists' choice.

Contingency management rewards desired behaviors, like adhering to treatment plans or managing symptoms. It can be combined with CBT to reinforce positive behaviors.

Dynamic psychotherapy explores unconscious thoughts, feelings, and motivations. Though less common for IBS, it may help those with psychological factors contributing to their symptoms, like unresolved trauma or emotional conflicts.

CBT for IBS can be tailored to individual needs and preferences, making it accessible to patients who may not have access to a specialist. Local support groups, hospitals, or clinics may also offer CBT programs.

Scientific evidence

CBT has proven effective for IBS, with studies showing significant improvements in symptoms and quality of life. Success rates range from 50-80%. CBT may be particularly beneficial for IBS patients experiencing anxiety or depression.

One large-scale study in 2020 analyzed 41 randomized controlled trials and found psychological therapies like CBT, gut-directed hypnotherapy, and relaxation therapy are effective in reducing IBS symptoms. Face-to-face and telephone-based CBT showed the best results.

So, why isn't CBT used more often? Some reasons include the following:

1. **Time commitment:** Most treatment plans last several months.
2. **Patient acceptance:** Not all patients may embrace psychotherapy or might prefer other treatments.
3. **Effectiveness:** CBT isn't a one-size-fits-all solution and may not work for everyone.
4. **Cost:** CBT can be expensive, and insurance may not cover it.

Despite these drawbacks, CBT remains a valuable treatment option for IBS.

Gut-directed hypnotherapy

Gut-directed hypnotherapy (GDH) is an exciting treatment that's been catching on for its potential to help IBS sufferers. This therapy uses hypnosis to tackle psychological or behavioral issues connected to IBS, aiming to relax people and manage their stress, which often plays a part in IBS symptoms.

GDH can help folks with IBS by:

- **Lowering stress and anxiety:** Hypnotherapy teaches relaxation techniques to ease the mind and reduce stress levels.
- **Tweaking the brain-gut connection:** Changing the communication between the brain and the gut, GDH might help ease IBS symptoms.
- **Boosting pain management:** Hypnotherapy helps individuals handle IBS-related pain.

How does GDH work?

Skilled hypnotherapists guide people through deep relaxation and visualization exercises in a series of sessions. Techniques involve creating a relaxed state and using suggestions to help manage symptoms. Individuals might also learn self-hypnosis for managing symptoms at home.

Scientific evidence

Several clinical trials have shown hypnotherapy can reduce IBS symptoms like abdominal pain, bloating, and diarrhea. For example:

- In 1984, a study reported that 71% of IBS patients who underwent GDH experienced symptom relief.
- Another study conducted in 2002 found that 12 sessions of GDH significantly improved the quality of life, anxiety levels, and IBS symptoms, with benefits lasting even up to a year later.
- In a 2023 study that used a smartphone app called Nerva to deliver GDH, 64% of patients reported a significant reduction in abdominal pain (>30%) after completing the program. Though adherence to the program was low, patients who completed all 42 sessions experienced notable improvements in their IBS symptoms. The study also revealed that patients aged 40 or older, who had been experiencing

symptoms for 5 years or more, may respond better to the app-delivered GDH.

While one-on-one treatment is the most effective form of hypnotherapy, there's solid evidence that virtual, group-based, or app-based treatments might also work. More research is needed on delivering hypnotherapy in these formats, making it easier and more affordable for patients in rural and urban areas to access treatment.

MBSR: Unraveling mindfulness for IBS relief

Mindfulness-based stress reduction (MBSR) is a structured program that helps folks deal with stress, pain, and other challenges. This technique uses mindfulness meditation, body awareness, and gentle yoga. MBSR has been helpful in managing various conditions, including IBS.

MBSR for IBS:

Stress and anxiety can worsen IBS symptoms, creating a cycle of discomfort and emotional upset. MBSR breaks this cycle by teaching people to focus on the present moment and become more aware of their thoughts, emotions, and physical sensations. This increased awareness helps IBS sufferers understand their triggers, manage stress, and respond better to symptoms.

Scientific evidence

Studies show MBSR can improve IBS symptoms, improve quality of life, and lower anxiety and depression. For example, a 2011 study found an 8-week MBSR program significantly improved IBS symptom severity and quality of life, with improvements lasting at a 3-month follow-up.

How to practice MBSR:

MBSR usually involves an 8-week group program led by a trained instructor. The program includes weekly 2.5-hour sessions and a day-long retreat. Participants are encouraged to practice mindfulness exercises daily for 30-45 minutes. The program covers the following:

- **Mindfulness meditation:** Learning to focus on breath and becoming aware of thoughts, feelings, and bodily sensations without judgment.

- **Body scan:** A guided meditation focusing sequentially on different body parts for awareness and relaxation.

- **Gentle yoga:** Simple stretching and yoga postures for body awareness and mindfulness.

Why consider GDPs, and where can you get them?

The 2021 American College of Gastroenterology's IBS management guidelines recommend gut-directed psychotherapies (GDPs) along with other treatments for emotionally stable patients whose thoughts and emotional patterns contribute to IBS symptoms.

GDP advantages:

- Safe when used by qualified professionals.
- Continued benefits even after stopping the therapy.
- Help patients with mixed-type IBS (IBS-M) or unclassified IBS (IBS-U) who have fewer medication options.

Resources for CBT:

- **Local support groups:** Organizations like the International Foundation for Gastrointestinal Disorders (IFFGD) can help find local groups that offer CBT or specialist referrals.

- **Local hospitals or clinics:** Inquire about CBT programs or specialist referrals at nearby hospitals or clinics.
- **Online therapy services:** Platforms like Talkspace, BetterHelp, and Amwell offer CBT for IBS with licensed therapists via video conferencing or messaging.
- **Telehealth options:** Many healthcare providers offer CBT sessions through telehealth.

Online therapy services and telehealth options make CBT more accessible to those without local specialists. Here are some resources for online therapy services and telehealth options:

- **Mahana for IBS:** https://www.mahana.com/treatments/ibs
- **BetterHelp:** https://www.betterhelp.com/
- **Talkspace:** https://www.talkspace.com/
- **Amwell:** https://amwell.com/
- **MDLive:** https://www.mdlive.com/
- **Psychology Today Therapist Directory:** https://www.psychologytoday.com/us/therapists
- **Open Path Psychotherapy Collective:** https://openpathcollective.org/
- **NAMI Mental Health Provider Directory:** https://www.nami.org/About-Mental-Illness/Treatments/Psychotherapy
- **BetterHelp Global:** https://www.betterhelp.com/global/
- **TherapyRoute:** https://www.therapyroute.com/
- **UK Council for Psychotherapy:** https://www.psychotherapy.org.uk/find-a-therapist/

GDP apps:

- **Mahana** (iOS, Android): A 12-week CBT program for IBS management.

No free trial. Costs $199/per 12-week program.

Pros: IBS-specific focus, FDA-cleared, clinically validated, prescription digital therapeutic CBT.

Cons: Expensive, limited to 12 weeks only.

- website: https://www.mahana.com/treatments/ibs
- iOS: https://apps.apple.com/us/app/mahana-ibs-treatment-relief/id1507233227
- Android: https://play.google.com/store/apps/details?id=com.mahana.android.app&hl=en_US&gl=US

- **Nerva** (iOS, Android): A 6-week gut-directed hypnotherapy program for IBS management using CBT principles.

  Offers a 7-day free trial, then a $59.99 3-month plan.

  Pros: IBS-specific focus, an evidence-based approach, and a credible developer.

  Cons: Limited free trial, subscription cost, and reliance on hypnotherapy.

  - website: https://try.nervaibs.com/
  - iOS: https://apps.apple.com/us/app/nerva-ibs-gut-hypnotherapy/id1467398796
  - Android: https://play.google.com/store/apps/details?id=com.mindsethealth.ibs&hl=en_US&gl=US

- **Zemedy** (iOS, Android): A personalized CBT program for IBS management.

  Offers a 7-day free trial, then $17.99/month or $89.99/year plans.

  Pro: IBS-specific focus and comprehensive symptom management.

  Cons: Subscription cost.

  - website: https://www.bold.health/

- iOS: https://apps.apple.com/us/app/zemedy-ibs-gut-health-care/id1442789941
- Android: https://play.google.com/store/apps/details?id=com.zemedyApp&hl=en_US&gl=US

Other Apps like Calm, Headspace, and Reachlink are not specific to IBS therapy but provide general mindfulness, meditation, and mental health support.

Summary of Gut-directed psychotherapies for IBS

Therapy Type	Description	Benefits	Limitations / Challenges
Cognitive-behavioral therapy (CBT)	A therapy addressing negative thought patterns and behaviors related to mental health issues, like anxiety and depression. It aims to help people identify and change unhelpful thoughts leading to negative emotions and behaviors.	- Can effectively address depression, anxiety disorders, eating disorders, and OCD - Improves IBS symptoms and quality of life	- Time commitment - Patient acceptance - Effectiveness varies - Cost (insurance may not cover)
Gut-directed hypnotherapy	A therapy using hypnosis to address psychological or behavioral issues connected to IBS, aiming to relax people and manage their stress.	- Lowers stress and anxiety - Improves brain-gut communication - Enhances pain management	- Requires skilled hypnotherapist - More research needed on alternative delivery formats

Mindfulness-based stress reduction (MBSR)	A structured program using mindfulness meditation, body awareness, and gentle yoga to help people deal with stress, pain, and other challenges.	- Reduces stress and anxiety - Improves IBS symptoms and quality of life - Enhances emotional well-being	- Requires commitment to an 8-week program - May require a trained instructor

Yoga for IBS: ancient wisdom for modern relief

Yoga, an ancient practice, combines physical poses, breathing exercises, and meditation to improve overall well-being. It has become popular as a complementary approach to managing various health conditions, including IBS. Let's dive into how yoga benefits IBS, the techniques involved, and the science backing it up.

Yoga helps IBS sufferers in several ways:

1. **Reducing stress:** Stress can trigger or worsen IBS symptoms. Yoga's focus on deep breathing and relaxation techniques calms the mind and eases stress, potentially alleviating IBS symptoms.
2. **Strengthening mind-body connection:** Yoga increases body awareness and response to different situations. This heightened awareness helps people identify and manage IBS triggers more effectively.
3. **Enhancing digestion and bowel function:** Some yoga poses are thought to improve digestion and promote regular bowel movements by gently massaging digestive organs.

Yoga for IBS involves physical postures (asanas), breathing exercises (pranayama), and relaxation or meditation techniques.

Some helpful poses for IBS sufferers include:

- Seated forward bend (Paschimottanasana)
- Wind-relieving pose (Pawanmuktasana)
- Bow pose (Dhanurasana)
- Cat-cow pose (Marjaryasana-Bitilasana)
- Bridge pose (Setu Bandhasana)

Scientific evidence

Scientific evidence supports yoga for IBS management. Studies show that yoga may be as effective as medications, CBT, exercise, and low FODMAP diets in reducing IBS symptoms, anxiety, depression, and stress. A study in 2015 showed that daily 1-hour yoga practice for 2 months significantly improved gastrointestinal symptoms, quality of life, and anxiety in IBS patients. Another study in 2016 study found that a 12-week yoga program significantly reduced IBS symptoms, anxiety, and stress compared to a control group receiving written self-care advice.

Keep in mind that individual responses to yoga can vary. If you're interested in trying yoga for IBS, consider joining a class or working with a certified yoga instructor familiar with IBS to guide you through appropriate poses and techniques.

Get moving: how exercise benefits IBS sufferers

Physical activity and exercise are vital for overall health and can help people with IBS. Regular exercise can ease IBS symptoms and boost overall well-being. Let's check out the potential benefits of exercise for IBS, how to add physical activity to your routine, and the science that backs it up.

Exercise benefits IBS sufferers in several ways

- **Reducing stress:** Stress can trigger or worsen IBS symptoms, and exercise is a natural way to lower stress levels. Physical activity releases endorphins, the body's "feel-good" chemicals, which ease stress and anxiety.
- **Improving bowel function:** Regular exercise stimulates digestive system muscles, promoting regular bowel movements and reducing the risk of constipation.
- **Enhancing overall well-being:** Exercise boosts mood, sleep quality, and energy levels, all affected by IBS.

To add exercise and physical activity to your routine, pick activities you enjoy and can easily fit into your daily schedule. Some examples of exercise for IBS include:

- walking
- swimming
- cycling
- yoga
- Pilates
- low-impact aerobics

Start slow and gradually crank up workout intensity and duration. Aim for at least 150 minutes of moderate-intensity exercise per week, as recommended by the American Heart Association.

Scientific evidence

A 2008 study showed that IBS patients participating in a 12-week moderate-intensity physical activity program experienced significant improvements in IBS symptoms, fatigue, and overall quality of life. Another study in 2011 found that IBS sufferers who did moderate to vigorous physical activity for 20-60 minutes three times per week for

12 weeks had significant symptom improvements compared to a control group getting general lifestyle advice.

Before starting a new exercise program, discuss it with a healthcare professional, especially if you have pre-existing conditions or concerns. They can help figure out the best exercise type and intensity for your specific needs, making sure you engage in physical activity safely and effectively.

Discover the magic of meditation for IBS relief

Did you know meditation can be a fantastic tool for managing IBS symptoms? It is true! This ancient practice that helps calm the mind and body can do wonders for those struggling with IBS.

Meditation works on IBS in several ways:

1. **Stress relief:** IBS symptoms often get worse with stress, but meditation can be a wonderful way to keep stress levels down. By calming the mind and body, you will find that IBS symptoms become more manageable.

2. **Mindful awareness:** Practicing meditation can increase awareness of your thoughts, emotions, and physical sensations. With greater mindfulness, you will better identify and manage IBS triggers.

3. **Balancing the gut-brain connection:** The gut and brain have a close relationship, which plays a significant role in IBS. Meditation can help regulate this connection, making it easier to deal with IBS symptoms.

So, how do you get started with meditation for IBS relief? It is easier than you think!

Just follow these simple steps:

- **Find a quiet, comfortable spot:** Choose a place to relax without distractions.
- **Set a timer:** Start with 5 to 10 minutes and gradually increase the duration as you get more comfortable with the practice.
- **Focus on your breath:** Close your eyes and concentrate on your breathing. Take deep breaths and exhale slowly, focusing on how your breath feels as it enters and leaves your body.
- **Observe your thoughts:** When your mind starts to wander (and it will), gently bring your focus back to your breath. It is natural for thoughts to come up during meditation but try to acknowledge them without judgment and then return your attention to your breath.
- **Practice regularly:** Consistency is key when it comes to experiencing the benefits of meditation. Aim to meditate every day, even if it is just for a few minutes.

Scientific evidence

Research findings have shown that meditation can be a powerful tool for managing IBS symptoms and improving overall well-being. For example, a study in 2011 found that an 8-week mindfulness-based program, which included meditation, significantly reduced IBS symptoms and improved participants' quality of life. These improvements lasted for at least three months after the program ended. Another study in 2013 discovered that meditation for just 8 weeks reduced IBS symptoms and improved overall psychological well-being.

Fast forward to 2015, yet another study found that IBS sufferers who practiced meditation and other mindfulness techniques experienced a significant decrease in IBS symptom severity and increased quality of life.

So, with its low risk and potential benefits, meditation is worth considering as a complementary approach to managing IBS symptoms. Remember, though, that everyone's response to meditation can be different. While it might work well for some, others may not experience the same benefits. Regardless, why not give meditation a try? It's a simple, cost-effective, and natural way to help manage IBS symptoms and promote a happier, more balanced life. Remember, practice makes perfect, so don't be too hard on yourself as you begin your meditation journey. Happy meditating!

Many Apps can help you practice meditation. Here are just a few:

Calm (iOS, Android) is a general meditation and mindfulness app that provides guided sessions to help users manage stress, anxiety, and sleep issues, which can indirectly benefit IBS sufferers.

Cost: 7-day free trial, followed by a subscription of $14.99/month, $69.99/year, or a one-time $ 399.99-lifetime purchase.

Pros: Wide range of content, customizable features, and accessibility to beginners and advanced users.

Cons: Not IBS-specific and subscription cost.

- website: https://www.calm.com/
- iOS: https://apps.apple.com/us/app/calm/id571800810
- Android: https://play.google.com/store/apps/details?id=com.calm.android

Headspace (iOS, Android) is a general meditation app that offers guided sessions to help users improve their mental well-being, reduce stress, and manage anxiety, which can indirectly benefit those with IBS.

Cost: 14-day free trial, followed by a $12.99/month subscription, $69.99/year, or a one-time $ 399.99-lifetime purchase.

Pros: User-friendly interface, variety of content, and suitable for beginners and experienced meditators.

Cons: Not IBS-specific and subscription cost.

- website: https://www.headspace.com/
- iOS: https://apps.apple.com/us/app/headspace-meditation-sleep/id493145008
- Android: https://play.google.com/store/apps/details?id=com.getsomeheadspace.android

CHAPTER 8

Managing IBS with Medications

"Drugs are not always necessary, but belief in recovery always is."
– Norman Cousins

D ealing with IBS can be a real struggle, especially when symptoms flare up. While changing your diet and managing stress can be helpful, sometimes it is just not enough. That is when medications and other treatments come into play. This section will discuss medications, including over the counter and prescription options.

The power and problem of a placebo

A placebo is a treatment or substance that has no therapeutic effect on a person's health. It is often used in clinical trials to compare the effectiveness of a new drug or therapy. Despite not containing active ingredients, placebos can sometimes cause real improvements in symptoms, known as the "placebo effect." The placebo effect results from the person's belief or expectation that the treatment will work.

Placebos are crucial in clinical trials because they allow researchers to compare the effectiveness of a real drug to something that shouldn't have any impact. The placebo effect has been observed in various conditions, including pain, depression, anxiety, and neurological disorders.

The use of placebos goes back to ancient times when healers would give patients sugar pills, herbs, or even animal parts as treatment. In the 18th century, they started being used in medical research to test new drugs. In clinical trials, patients are divided into groups receiving the actual drug or a placebo. The placebo group often improves, indicating that belief in treatment can make a significant difference in our health.

An interesting story from the 1950s shows the power of placebos. Researchers at the Mayo Clinic were testing a new blood pressure medication called Reserpine. They found that patients who took a placebo also had reduced blood pressure, much like those who received the actual drug. The researchers discovered that the placebo tablets had a bitter taste, which patients associated with the drug's efficacy. This association led them to believe that the placebo was working, and their belief played a crucial role in their improvement.

The exact mechanism of placebos is still unclear, but it may be related to endorphins and other brain chemicals. Given the close connection between the brain and gut, placebos can be particularly effective for IBS. Studies have shown that if given a sugar pill for IBS symptoms and if a person believes that it works, there is a 40% chance of symptom relief. This illustrates the power of the mind and expectations in influencing a person's experience of treatment outcomes.

A study published in 2009 using Amitriptyline to relieve IBS symptoms in children showed that 63% of patients experienced an improvement in the Amitriptyline group. Amazingly, 57.5% of patients who received a placebo also reported feeling better! Since placebos work so well for IBS, it can be challenging for drug companies to prove in clinical trials that their medications are even better than placebos. Nonetheless, many medication options are still available for managing IBS.

Over-the-counter medications and supplements for IBS

Over the counter (OTC) medications can help with specific IBS symptoms like diarrhea, constipation, and bloating. Here are some common OTC medications for IBS, but always follow package instructions or your doctor's advice.

Laxatives:

Laxatives can help people with constipation symptoms of IBS, but they may not help with other symptoms like abdominal pain.

How OTC laxatives work

OTC laxatives are grouped into categories based on how they work:

- Osmotic laxatives attract water into the intestines, softening the stool and making it easier to pass.
- Stimulant laxatives speed up intestinal movement, encouraging bowel movements.

Common OTC laxatives

- Osmotic laxatives: Polyethylene glycol (MiraLAX), magnesium hydroxide (Milk of Magnesia)
- Stimulant laxatives: Bisacodyl (Dulcolax), sennosides (Senokot)

Usual dosages

- Polyethylene glycol (MiraLAX): A typical dosage is 17 grams mixed with water, taken once a day.
- Magnesium hydroxide: The suggested dosage is 2-4 tablespoons taken once a day.

- Bisacodyl (Dulcolax): A standard adult dosage is 5-15 mg, taken once a day.
- Sennosides (Senokot): The recommended dosage is 15-30 mg, taken once a day.

Side effects

- Osmotic laxatives: Bloating, gas, diarrhea, electrolyte imbalance (with excessive use)
- Stimulant laxatives: Abdominal cramping and diarrhea.

Scientific evidence

- Osmotic laxatives: Polyethylene glycol is proven to help with constipation in IBS patients. Long-term studies show that it's more effective than other OTC or even some prescription laxatives and is well-tolerated over time.
- Stimulant laxatives: They are safe long-term and have proven effective in treating constipation. Both senna and bisacodyl may need a dose adjustment if they cause abdominal pain and diarrhea. Senna is generally better tolerated compared to bisacodyl.

If you're looking for a safe and effective laxative for long-term use, I suggest trying MiraLAX or Senna. Don't be concerned about the misconception that long-term use of laxatives can lead to dependence or harm your colon, as it is not true. However, if you are struggling with constipation related to IBS, stool softeners may not be the best option.

Anti-diarrheal medications

Anti-diarrheals may not help other symptoms of IBS, like abdominal pain or bloating. They help reduce bowel movement frequency to make your life more manageable and predictable, especially when you go outside or when you are traveling.

How do they work?

OTC anti-diarrheal medications mainly slow down your intestines. This gives your body more time to soak up water from the stool, making it firmer and easier to manage.

Popular OTC anti-diarrheals

- Loperamide (Imodium)

- Bismuth subsalicylate (Pepto-Bismol, Kaopectate)

Typical dosages

Loperamide: Adults usually start with 2 mg every 6 hours. Don't take more than 8 mg per day.

Bismuth subsalicylate: Adults usually take 2 tablets or 30 mL of liquid every 30-60 minutes, but no more than 8 doses in 24 hours.

Possible side effects

Loperamide: Watch out for dizziness, drowsiness, constipation, and abdominal pain.

Bismuth subsalicylate: You might experience darkened stools or tongue, mild constipation, and nausea.

Scientific evidence

Loperamide: Research shows loperamide effectively reduces diarrhea in IBS patients, but it may not improve other IBS symptoms.

Bismuth subsalicylate: There's limited evidence for its effectiveness in IBS-related diarrhea, but it is commonly used for general diarrhea relief.

To sum up, OTC anti-diarrheals like loperamide and bismuth subsalic-ylate can help you manage diarrhea caused by IBS. While loperamide is backed by research, the evidence for bismuth subsalicylate is limited.

Fiber supplements

Fiber supplements can help reduce constipation for people with IBS-C. Let's explore how fiber supplements work, their common types, dosag-es, side effects, and what science says about their effectiveness.

How do fiber supplements work?

There are two kinds of fiber- soluble and insoluble. Soluble fiber dis-solves in water and creates a gel-like substance, softening stools and regulating bowel movements. Insoluble fiber doesn't dissolve in water and adds bulk to stools, helping constipation. Soluble fiber is proven to be more effective in easing IBS symptoms.

The exact reason why fiber helps IBS isn't fully known. One theory suggests that psyllium increases short-chain fatty acid production like butyrate, which might have anti-inflammatory effects on the colon lin-ing. Another possibility is that soluble fiber could change gut bacteria balance, contributing to its positive effects on IBS symptoms.

Popular OTC soluble fiber supplements

- Psyllium (Metamucil, Konsyl)
- Methylcellulose (Citrucel)
- Wheat dextrin (Benefiber)

Typical dosages

Psyllium: Adults usually take 1-2 teaspoons mixed with 8 oz (240mL) of water up to 3 times a day.

Methylcellulose: Adults typically use 1-2 tablespoons mixed with 8 oz (240mL) of water up to 3 times a day.

Wheat dextrin: Adults typically take 1-2 teaspoons mixed with 4-8 oz (120-240mL) of water up to 3 times daily.

Possible side effects

Psyllium: Watch out for bloating, gas, and stomach cramps. Drink plenty of water to avoid digestive problems.

Methylcellulose: Side effects include bloating, gas, and stomach cramps. Make sure to drink enough water when taking methylcellulose.

Wheat dextrin: You might experience bloating, gas, and abdominal discomfort.

Scientific evidence

Psyllium: Research shows that psyllium improves IBS symptoms, including constipation and diarrhea, compared to a placebo.

Methylcellulose and Wheat dextrin: There's limited research on methylcellulose and wheat dextrin for IBS, but they are widely used for constipation relief and promoting bowel regularity.

To sum up, taking OTC fiber supplements such as psyllium, methylcellulose, and wheat dextrin can be beneficial for people with IBS who experience mild constipation. Psyllium has been found to be effective in relieving IBS symptoms, although further research is necessary for methylcellulose and wheat dextrin. If you suffer from severe constipation, it is recommended to use laxatives such as polyethylene glycol or Senna, or bisacodyl instead of fiber supplements.

Gas-relieving medications for IBS

Bloating and gas can really put a damper on your day when you have IBS. But don't worry. Gas-relieving medications are coming to the rescue! *See Chapter 10 for a more detailed discussion on the management of bloating.*

How do gas-relieving medications work?

These medications, also known as anti-gas or anti-flatulence agents, break up gas bubbles in your digestive system. Those annoying bubbles cause discomfort and make you feel bloated. By smashing the bubbles, the medications help release trapped gas, so your body can get rid of it more easily.

Popular gas-relieving medications

- Simethicone: It changes the surface tension of gas bubbles, making them combine into larger bubbles that are easier to expel from your body.
- Activated Charcoal: This is believed to absorb excess gas in your gut, reducing bloating and gas.

Common dosages

Simethicone: Adults typically take 40-125 mg after meals and at bedtime, as needed. The dose can be repeated up to four times a day.

Activated Charcoal: Adults usually take 500-1000 mg after meals as needed.

Side effects

Simethicone: Since the body does not absorb it, simethicone has few side effects. Rarely, some people might experience mild side effects like diarrhea or nausea.

Activated Charcoal: Watch out for dark stools, constipation, and, rarely, vomiting.

Scientific evidence

Simethicone: While it is widely used for gas relief, scientific evidence supporting its effectiveness in IBS is limited. Some studies suggest that it may help with gas and bloating, but more research is needed.

Activated charcoal: A small study showed that activated charcoal might help reduce gas production and bloating in IBS patients. However, more extensive and high-quality research is needed to confirm these results.

In conclusion, gas-relieving medications like simethicone and activated charcoal might help with IBS-related bloating and gas. However, more research is needed to confirm their effectiveness. Remember that while these agents can provide temporary relief, they don't treat the underlying cause of IBS.

Category	Medication	Mechanism of Action	Dosage	Common Side Effects	Used For
Laxatives	Polyethylene glycol (MiraLAX)	Osmotic laxative: Attracts water into intestines	17 grams mixed with water once a day	Bloating, gas, diarrhea, electrolyte imbalance	IBS-related constipation
	Magnesium hydroxide (Milk of Magnesia)	Osmotic laxative: Attracts water into intestines	2-4 tablespoons, once a day	Bloating, gas, diarrhea, electrolyte imbalance	IBS-related constipation
	Bisacodyl (Dulcolax)	Stimulant laxative: Speeds up intestinal movement	5-15 mg, once a day	Abdominal cramping, diarrhea	IBS-related constipation

	Sennosides (Senokot)	Stimulant laxative: Speeds up intestinal movement	15-30 mg, once a day	Abdominal cramping, diarrhea	IBS-related constipation
Anti-diarrheals	Loperamide (Imodium)	Slows down intestines	4 mg initially, 2 mg after each loose stool, and up to 8 mg per day	Dizziness, drowsiness, constipation, abdominal pain	IBS-related diarrhea
	Bismuth subsalicylate (Pepto-Bismol, Kaopectate)	Slows down intestines	2 tablets or 30 mL every 30-60 minutes, up to 8 doses in 24 hours	Darkened stools or tongue, mild constipation, nausea	IBS-related diarrhea
Fiber Supplements	Psyllium (Metamucil, Konsyl)	Soluble fiber: Dissolves in water, softens stools	1-2 teaspoons mixed with water, up to 3 times a day	Bloating, gas, stomach cramps	IBS-C constipation relief
	Methylcellulose (Citrucel)	Soluble fiber: Dissolves in water, softens stools	1-2 tablespoons mixed with water, up to 3 times a day	Bloating, gas, stomach cramps	IBS-C constipation relief
	Wheat dextrin (Benefiber)	Soluble fiber: Dissolves in water, softens stools	2 teaspoons mixed with water, up to 3 times a day	Bloating, gas, abdominal discomfort	IBS-C constipation relief
Gas-Relieving Medications	Simethicone	Breaks up gas bubbles in the digestive system	40-125 mg after meals and at bedtime, up to 4 times a day	Mild side effects like diarrhea or nausea (rare)	IBS-related bloating and gas
	Activated Charcoal	Absorbs excess gas in the gut	500-1000 mg after meals as needed	Dark stools, constipation, vomiting (rare)	IBS-related bloating and gas

Medications to treat overall IBS symptoms

Antispasmodics

How do they work?

Antispasmodics relax the muscles in your gut and relieve the cramps and spasms that come with IBS.

Antispasmodic medications:

1. **Dicyclomine (Bentyl)**

Dosage: Usually 10-20 mg, four times daily, before meals and bedtime (maximum daily dose: 160 mg). Always follow your doctor's advice.

   Side effects: Dry mouth, blurry vision, dizziness, drowsiness, constipation, trouble peeing, and nausea.

2. **Hyoscyamine (Levsin)**

Dosage: Usually 0.125-0.25 mg, every four hours as needed. Always follow your doctor's advice.

   Side Effects: Dry mouth, blurry vision, dizziness, drowsiness, constipation, faster heart rate, and trouble peeing.

3. **Phenobarbital, hyoscyamine, atropine, and scopolamine (Donnatal)**

Dosage: Usually 1-2 tablets or 5 mL elixir, three to four times daily. The dosage depends on symptom severity.

   Side effects: Dry mouth, blurry vision, dizziness, drowsiness, constipation, faster heart rate, and trouble peeing.

4. **Methscopolamine bromide (Pamine)**

Dosage: Usually 2.5-5 mg, three to four times daily, before meals and bedtime. Always follow your doctor's advice.

Side Effects: Dry mouth, blurry vision, dizziness, drowsiness, constipation, faster heart rate, and trouble peeing.

5. **Probanthine (propantheline bromide)**

Dosage: Usually 7.5-15 mg, three to four times daily, before meals and bedtime.

Side effects: Dry mouth, blurry vision, dizziness, drowsiness, constipation, faster heart rate, and trouble peeing.

Scientific evidence

A review of 22 studies with 1,778 patients using 12 antispasmodic drugs showed that antispasmodics were more effective than placebos. Levsin stood out as particularly effective. Other medications like Otilonium and Cometropoum, which aren't FDA-approved for IBS in the US, also showed promise.

However, the research has its limitations. The studies aren't of the highest quality, making comparisons difficult. There might be a bias toward publishing only positive results, and few studies have been done on each specific antispasmodic.

Nonetheless, antispasmodics can be helpful on a selective basis. They may help someone with uncomfortable abdominal cramping, particularly if they have already tried diet and lifestyle changes but aren't keen on antidepressants.

Antidepressants

Tricyclic Antidepressants (TCAs): not just for depression

TCAs were made to treat depression, but surprise! They can help with IBS too. By boosting brain chemicals like serotonin and norepinephrine, they can improve mood and gut function.

Some commonly used TCAs:

- Desipramine
- Nortriptyline
- Amitriptyline

Dosage: Lower than for depression, for example, 10-25 mg of amitriptyline, whereas for depression, doses as high as 150-200mg per day are used.

Side effects: Dry mouth, drowsiness, blurred vision, constipation, and trouble urinating. Due to the side effects of drowsiness, it is recommended to use it at bedtime.

Selective Serotonin Reuptake Inhibitors (SSRIs): serotonin superstars

SSRIs also help IBS by raising serotonin levels in the brain, which can improve mood, pain, and gut function.

Some commonly used SSRIs:

- Fluoxetine
- Sertraline
- Paroxetine

Dosage: Depends upon the SSRI. For example, 20 mg of fluoxetine once a day. Your doctor will decide the right amount for you.

Side effects: Nausea, diarrhea, headache, insomnia, and drowsiness.

SSRIs vs. SNRIs for IBS: what's the difference?

SSRIs increase serotonin, while SNRIs raise serotonin and norepinephrine. Both brain chemicals help regulate mood and pain. Some common SNRIs include duloxetine (Cymbalta), venlafaxine (Effexor XR), and desvenlafaxine (Pristiq).

Scientific evidence

- TCAs: A study of 14 trials found TCAs improved IBS symptoms and abdominal pain. They're especially helpful for IBS-D (diarrhea) and IBS-M (mixed) types.
- SSRIs: According to a review of 12 trials, SSRIs were found to be helpful in relieving IBS symptoms, but more high-quality research is needed.
- SNRIs: Limited research, but a small 2016 study suggested duloxetine (Cymbalta) could reduce pain and improve life quality in IBS patients.

TCAs are generally more effective than SSRIs or SNRIs for IBS. However, since TCAs can cause constipation, SSRIs might be better for IBS-C.

Combination Drugs:

Librax

Librax combines chlordiazepoxide (a benzodiazepine) and clidinium bromide (an antispasmodic). It treats IBS by easing abdominal pain, cramps, and spasms.

How does Librax work?

Chlordiazepoxide reduces anxiety and stress, while clidinium bromide relaxes the gut's smooth muscles to lessen spasms and discomfort.

Dosage: Usually 1-2 capsules, three to four times daily, before meals and bedtime. Follow your doctor's advice.

Side effects: Drowsiness, dizziness, dry mouth, blurred vision, constipation, trouble urinating, nausea, and weakness. Librax can also cause dependence and withdrawal symptoms.

Librax is preferred for those with both functional dyspepsia and IBS, as it is effective for upper and lower GI symptoms.

Category	Medication	Mechanism of Action	Dosage	Common Side Effects	Used For
A. Antispasmodics*	Dicyclomine (Bentyl)	Calms intestinal muscles and relieves cramps and spasms	10-20 mg, four times a day, before meals and bedtime	*See below	IBS-D, IBS-C
	Hyoscyamine (Levsin)	Calms intestinal muscles and relieves cramps and spasms	0.125-0.25 mg, every four hours as needed	*See below	IBS-D, IBS-C
	Phenobarbital, hyoscyamine, atropine, and scopolamine (Donnatal)	Calms intestinal muscles and relieves cramps and spasms	1-2 tablets or 5 mL elixir, three to four times daily	*See below	IBS-D, IBS-C
	Methscopolamine bromide (Pamine)	Calms intestinal muscles and relieves cramps and spasms	2.5-5 mg, three to four times daily, before meals and bedtime	*See below	IBS-D, IBS-C
	Propantheline bromide (Probanthine)	Calms intestinal muscles and relieves cramps and spasms	7.5-15 mg, three to four times daily, before meals and bedtime	*See below	IBS-D, IBS-C
B. Antidepressants (TCAs)	Desipramine, Nortriptyline, Amitriptyline	Boost brain chemicals like serotonin and norepinephrine to improve mood and gut function	Lower than for depression, e.g., 10-25 mg of amitriptyline at bedtime	Dry mouth, drowsiness, blurred vision, constipation, trouble urinating	IBS
B. Antidepressants (SSRIs)	Fluoxetine, Sertraline, Paroxetine	Raise serotonin levels in the brain to improve mood, pain, and gut function	Depends on the SSRI, e.g., 20 mg of fluoxetine once a day	Nausea, diarrhea, headache, insomnia, drowsiness	IBS

C. Combination Drugs	Librax (chlordiazepoxide and clidinium bromide)	Reduces anxiety and stress, relaxes gut's smooth muscles	1-2 capsules, three to four times a day, before meals and bedtime	Drowsiness, dizziness, dry mouth, blurred vision, constipation, trouble urinating, nausea, weakness	IBS, Functional dyspepsia

*Common Side Effects for Antispasmodics: Dry mouth, blurry vision, dizziness, drowsiness, constipation, faster heart rate, and trouble peeing.

Prescription medications to treat IBS-C

These drugs help by increasing fluid in the intestines, which improves bowel movements and eases constipation. However, these medications are not just laxatives. They also help with other symptoms of IBS, like abdominal pain and bloating.

Some of the approved drugs for IBS-C treatment: Linaclotide (Linzess), Lubiprostone (Amitiza), Plecanatide (Trulance), and Tenapanor (IBSrela).

Usual dosages:
- Linzess: 290 mcg once daily on an empty stomach for adults.
- Amitiza: 8 mcg twice daily with food for adult women.
- Trulance: 3 mg once daily for adults.
- Ibsrela: 50 mg twice daily for adults.

Side effects:
- Linzess: Diarrhea, belly pain, gas, and bloating.
- Amitiza: Nausea, diarrhea, headache, and belly pain.
- Trulance: Diarrhea, belly pain, and gas.

- Ibsrela: Diarrhea, abdominal distension, and gas.

Scientific evidence:

- Linzess: In a 26-week study with 804 IBS-C patients, 34% of Linzess users saw improvements in bowel movement frequency and belly pain, compared to 14% on placebo.

- Amitiza: Two studies involving 1,154 IBS-C patients showed that 18% of Amitiza users saw improvements in bowel movement frequency and consistency, compared to 10% on placebo. Amitiza worked better for women than men.

- Trulance: A 12-week study with 1,054 IBS-C patients found that 30% of Trulance users experienced improvements in constipation and belly pain, compared to 18% on placebo.

- Ibsrela: In a 26-week study with 603 IBS-C patients, 36% on Tenapanor saw improvements in bowel movement frequency and belly pain, compared to 23% on placebo.

In a nutshell, all these drugs effectively treat overall IBS-C symptoms, not just constipation. They work quickly, and their effects last over time. Diarrhea is the most common side effect, but it's generally mild, and the drugs are well tolerated.

Category	Medication	Mechanism of Action	Dosage	Common Side Effects	Used For
Prescription Medications for IBS-C	Linaclotide (Linzess)	Increases fluid in the intestines, improving bowel movements	290 mcg once daily on an empty stomach for adults	Diarrhea, belly pain, gas, bloating	IBS-C
	Lubiprostone (Amitiza)	Increases fluid in the intestines, improving bowel movements	8 mcg twice daily with food for adult women	Nausea, diarrhea, headache, belly pain	IBS-C
	Plecanatide (Trulance)	Increases fluid in the intestines, improving bowel movements	3 mg once daily for adults	Diarrhea, belly pain, gas	IBS-C
	Tenapanor (IBSrela)	Increases fluid in the intestines, improving bowel movements	50 mg twice daily for adults	Diarrhea, abdominal distension, gas	IBS-C

Prescription Medications to Treat IBS-D

Viberzi, Xifaxan, and Lotronex are FDA-approved medications to treat IBS-D.

Viberzi (Eluxadoline)

How it works: Viberzi activates specific gut receptors called opioid receptors. This slows down food movement in the digestive system, reducing diarrhea and abdominal pain in people with IBS-D.

Dosage: Viberzi is usually taken in doses of 75 mg or 100 mg twice daily with food.

Side effects:

- Constipation
- Nausea

125

- Abdominal pain
- Gas or bloating

Scientific evidence:

In a 2016 study with 2,428 IBS-D patients, 33% taking Viberzi saw improvements in abdominal pain and stool consistency compared to 20% on placebo. Viberzi was generally well-tolerated, with constipation being the most common side effect. This medication is not recommended if you have had your gallbladder removed.

Xifaxan (Rifaximin)

How it works: Xifaxan is an antibiotic that targets gut bacteria. It helps IBS-D by reducing harmful bacteria and improving the bacterial balance in the intestines.

Dosage: Xifaxan's usual dosage for IBS-D is 550 mg, taken three times daily for 14 days.

Side effects:

- Nausea
- Gas or bloating
- Headache

Scientific evidence:

A large trial with 1,260 IBS-D patients showed Xifaxan (550 mg) taken three times daily for 14 days improved bloating and overall IBS symptoms in 40% of patients compared to 30% on placebo.

Lotronex (Alosetron): the last resort for severe IBS-D in women

How it works: Lotronex blocks serotonin receptors in the gut, slowing down food movement in the digestive system. It is used specifically to treat IBS-D in women who haven't responded to other treatments.

Dosage: The usual starting dosage of Lotronex is 0.5 mg, taken twice daily. If needed, the dose can be increased to 1 mg twice daily.

Side effects:

- Constipation
- Gas or bloating
- Nausea
- Reduced blood flow to the intestines causing colitis is rare

Scientific evidence:

Clinical trials show Lotronex can effectively reduce abdominal pain, urgency, and diarrhea in women with IBS-D. However, due to potentially severe side effects, its use is restricted and prescribed only to those who have not found relief with other treatments. The current evidence supports using Alosetron (Lotronex) *only* in women with severe IBS-D when other interventions have failed.

Category	Medication	Mechanism of Action	Dosage	Common Side Effects	Used For
Prescription Medications for IBS-D	Rifaximin (Xifaxan)	Reduces gut bacteria overgrowth and lowers inflammation	550 mg, taken three times daily for 14 days	Nausea, gas, bloating, headache	IBS-D
	Eluxadoline (Viberzi)	Activates opioid receptors in the gut to slow down food movement	75 mg or 100 mg, twice daily with food	Constipation, nausea, abdominal pain, gas, bloating	IBS-D (Not recommended for someone who had their gallbladder removed)
	Alosetron (Lotronex)	Blocks serotonin receptors in the gut to slow down food movement	0.5 mg, taken twice daily; can be increased to 1 mg twice daily if needed	Constipation, gas, bloating, nausea, rare severe side effects	Severe IBS-D in women

Choosing the proper IBS medication: a personalized approach

When to use medication?

As a medical professional, my first priority is to recommend diet and lifestyle changes to my patients before suggesting medication. If these changes are not effective or do not work at all, I will have open and thorough discussions with my patients about different medication options. During these discussions, I provide detailed information about the benefits, drawbacks, and potential side effects of each medication, as well as any cost and insurance coverage considerations that may apply in the United States.

For mild symptoms: When dealing with mild symptoms such as occasional abdominal pain, I typically prescribe peppermint oil capsules (*discussed in the next chapter*) alongside dietary changes. Alternatively, I may suggest an anti-spasmodic medication that can be taken as needed for quick pain relief.

For daily symptoms: For patients experiencing daily symptoms that require long-term maintenance medication, I often recommend tricyclic antidepressants.

For overlapping functional dyspepsia: In these cases, I prefer using Librax or tricyclic antidepressants.

For severe symptoms: I may prescribe newer medications such as Linzess or Trulance for IBS-C while Viberzi or Xifaxan are suitable choices for IBS-D.

For bloating as the main symptom: If a patient's primary concern is bloating, I may use Xifaxan or similar antibiotics, as they are short-term medications. These are preferred by patients who don't want to be on long-term medications.

There are numerous medication options available to treat severe IBS symptoms. However, the specific choice depends on individual factors and will be customized to each patient's needs. While this medications section provides a general overview of available options for IBS, it is not a replacement for proper medical advice from your doctor. Your doctor can assist with selecting the appropriate medication, dosages, and other recommendations discussed in this chapter.

CHAPTER 9

Complementary and Alternative Treatments

"The art of healing comes from nature, not from the physician. There-fore, the physician must start from nature, with an open mind."
– Paracelsus

Complementary treatments are types of therapies that can be used along with conventional medical treatments, while alternative treatments are used in place of conventional treatments. The goal of both is to alleviate symptoms and enhance one's quality of life. Let's explore some common complementary and alternative treatments for IBS.

1. Peppermint oil

Peppermint oil, from the peppermint plant, has been a go-to natural remedy for digestive issues. Its main ingredient, menthol, relaxes the gastrointestinal tract's smooth muscles, easing spasms and discomfort.

Scientific evidence

Research supports peppermint oil's effectiveness in easing IBS symptoms. A meta-analysis of nine clinical trials found significant improvements compared to a placebo. In addition, a 2019 review of twelve studies suggested that it is a safe and effective short-term option for IBS.

How to use peppermint oil

Enteric-coated capsules ensure peppermint oil reaches the intestines. Follow the recommended dosage on the packaging and consult your healthcare provider before starting any new supplement.

2. Iberogast®

Iberogast® is an herbal supplement with nine plant extracts, including peppermint, chamomile, and caraway. It is thought to have anti-inflammatory, antispasmodic, and gut-regulating properties.

Scientific evidence

A meta-analysis of five clinical trials found Iberogast® significantly improved IBS symptoms and abdominal pain compared to a placebo. Another study of 208 patients found it to be more effective than a placebo in reducing IBS symptoms after four weeks.

How to use Iberogast®

Iberogast® comes in liquid form and can be taken with or without meals. Follow the recommended dosage on the packaging and consult your healthcare provider before starting any new supplement.

3. Caraway oil

Caraway oil, from caraway plant seeds, has traditionally been used to relieve digestive discomfort. It is believed to have antispasmodic and carminative (helps relieve gas) properties that may help reduce intestinal spasms and gas.

Scientific evidence

While limited studies exist on caraway oil for IBS, its combination with peppermint oil has shown promise. A study found this combination effectively reduced IBS symptoms compared to a placebo.

How to use Caraway oil

Caraway oil comes in capsule and oil forms. The dosage varies depending upon the formulation but typically ranges from 0.2-2 mL per dose, up to three times daily. Follow the recommended dosage on the product label and take it with food to avoid stomach irritation.

4. Fecal microbiota transplantation (FMT)

Imagine a treatment for IBS that is a little out of the ordinary: transplanting poop from a healthy person into the gut of someone with IBS. It is called fecal microbiota transplantation (FMT). It might just be the key to restoring gut balance for some IBS sufferers.

Scientific evidence

A paper published in 2023 reviewed 12 clinical trials conducted between 2017 and 2021 and found promising results for FMT as a potential solution for IBS patients. While a meta-analysis of 7 randomized controlled trials with 489 participants showed that FMT did not improve IBS symptoms overall, it did demonstrate potential benefits for individuals with constipation-related IBS.

Post-infectious IBS

In 2022, a study discovered that FMT could be particularly beneficial for patients with post-infectious IBS (PI-IBS). Nevertheless, there are still numerous unanswered questions. We need to find out if this treatment works better than just giving a placebo, like using the patient's own poop, fake pills, or just cleaning out their bowels. We also need to figure out who the best stool donor is, how often we should do the treatment, the right amount to use, and the best way to give it to the patient.

FMT's future in IBS treatment

At the moment, FMT is not a recommended treatment for IBS. But there is a lot of excitement around its potential, especially for specific groups of IBS patients.

5. Probiotics

Probiotics are live microorganisms, like bacteria and yeasts, that keep us healthy when consumed in the right amounts.

How do probiotics work?

These live microorganisms maintain a healthy balance in your gut. They help IBS by improving gut function, boosting the gut barrier, and reducing inflammation.

Common probiotic supplements

Some common probiotics for IBS include Lactobacillus, Bifidobacterium, and Saccharomyces boulardii.

Scientific evidence

One large-scale study combining data from 43 clinical trials showed that probiotics improved IBS symptoms in 21% of patients. Another review looked at 35 trials with 3452 IBS patients and found that specific probiotics, like Bifidobacterium and certain combos, helped with symptoms like tummy pain and bloating. But here's the catch: we still don't know which exact probiotics are the best because each study used different mixes.

Usual dosages

Dosages depend on the specific strain and product. A standard recommendation is 10-50 billion colony-forming units (CFUs) per day. Always follow package instructions.

Side effects

Most people handle probiotics well, but some may experience side effects like gas, bloating, or upset stomach. These side effects usually go away as your body adjusts to the supplement.

6. Prebiotics

Prebiotics are non-digestible fibers that can assist the beneficial bacteria in our gut. Both probiotics and prebiotics can help improve gut health and reduce IBS symptoms.

How do prebiotics work?

Prebiotics are a type of fiber that may improve gut health and alleviate IBS symptoms by nourishing the good bacteria.

Common prebiotic supplements

Popular prebiotics include inulin, fructooligosaccharides (FOS), and galactooligosaccharides (GOS).

Scientific evidence

Research on prebiotics for IBS is limited. A small study found that taking a GOS supplement improved IBS symptoms. However, more research is needed to confirm these findings.

Usual dosages

The recommended daily intake for prebiotics is usually around 5-20 grams. As with probiotics, follow the package instructions or your doctor's recommendations.

Side effects

Potential side effects of prebiotics include gas, bloating, and stomach cramps. To minimize these side effects, start with a low dose and gradually increase it over time.

7. Acupuncture

Acupuncture, a traditional Chinese medicine technique involving the insertion of thin needles into specific points on the body, has been used for thousands of years to treat various health conditions, including digestive issues.

Scientific evidence

A study from 2021 combined the results of 61 clinical trials to see if acupuncture works for digestive issues like IBS. Results show that this treatment is more effective than others and has fewer negative side effects.

Another study in 2022 looked at the data from 24 clinical trials that included 2151 patients, to check if acupuncture could ease the emotional rollercoaster that comes with IBS. Guess what? Acupuncture beats medications in calming down anxiety and depression in IBS patients. But it is still a bit of a mystery if it is the placebo effect or if it genuinely works. We need more research to confirm these results and find the best acupuncture method. Still, it is worth considering, especially for those tough-to-treat IBS cases.

How to try acupuncture

If you want acupuncture for IBS management, consult your healthcare provider for recommendations and referrals to qualified acupuncturists.

8. Chinese herbal medicine

A meta-analysis of 10 studies involving 2500 patients showed that Chinese herbal medicine worked better than the usual IBS treatments. But more research is needed to know how safe and effective these herbal remedies are.

9. Ginger

Ginger, a popular spice, and traditional remedy has been used for centuries to soothe digestive issues. It is believed to have anti-inflammatory and antispasmodic properties, making it a potential option for IBS symptom relief.

Scientific evidence

While there is limited research on ginger for IBS, a study found ginger supplements significantly reduced IBS severity in patients compared to a placebo. More research is needed to confirm these findings and establish the optimal dosage.

How to use ginger

Ginger comes in various forms, including capsules, teas, and fresh or powdered root. Follow the recommended dosage on the packaging and consult your healthcare provider before starting any new supplement.

10. Licorice Root

Licorice root, from the Glycyrrhiza glabra plant, has been used in traditional medicine to treat gastrointestinal issues. It is believed to have anti-inflammatory and soothing properties that may benefit IBS sufferers.

Scientific evidence

There is limited research on licorice root for IBS. Some studies have explored its use in treating other gastrointestinal issues, but more research is needed to establish its efficacy and safety for IBS patients.

How to use licorice root

Licorice root comes in various forms, including teas, capsules, and chewable tablets. Follow the recommended dosage on the packaging and consult your healthcare provider before starting any new supplement.

11. Fennel

Fennel, a flavorful herb with a licorice-like taste, has been used in traditional medicine to address digestive issues. It is believed to have antispasmodic, carminative (helps relieve gas), and anti-inflammatory properties, which may help alleviate IBS symptoms.

Scientific evidence

Research on fennel for IBS is limited, but a study found that combining fennel and curcumin effectively reduced IBS symptoms and improved quality of life. More research will determine fennel's optimal dosage and long-term effects for IBS management.

How to use fennel

Fennel comes in various forms, including teas, capsules, and seeds. Follow the recommended dosage on the packaging and consult your healthcare provider before starting any new supplement.

12. Slippery elm

Slippery elm, derived from the inner bark of the slippery elm tree, has traditionally been used to soothe the digestive system. Its soluble fiber, called mucilage, forms a gel-like substance when mixed with water, which can help protect and soothe the gut's lining.

Scientific evidence

While limited research specifically focuses on slippery elm for IBS, its soothing properties have been acknowledged in traditional medicine. More research is needed to fully understand its effectiveness in IBS management.

How to use slippery elm

Slippery elm comes in various forms, including capsules, powders, and teas. Follow the recommended dosage on the packaging and consult your healthcare provider before starting any new supplement.

13. Artichoke leaf extract

Artichoke leaf extract, from the leaves of the globe artichoke plant, has been used for centuries to support digestive health. It stimulates bile production, aiding fat digestion and positively affecting gut motility.

Scientific evidence

A study involving 208 IBS patients found that artichoke leaf extract significantly reduced IBS symptoms and improved quality of life compared to a placebo over six weeks. More research is needed to confirm these findings and determine the optimal dosage for IBS management.

How to use artichoke leaf extract

Artichoke leaf extract comes in capsule form. Follow the recommended dosage on the packaging and consult your healthcare provider before starting any new supplement.

14. Aloe Vera

Aloe vera, known for its skin-soothing properties, has also been used to support digestive health. The gel inside the leaves contains vitamins, minerals, and enzymes that can help reduce inflammation and promote gut healing.

Scientific evidence

There is limited research on the effectiveness of aloe vera for IBS. While some anecdotal reports suggest it may help relieve IBS symptoms, more scientific studies are needed to establish its efficacy and safety.

How to use aloe vera

Aloe vera comes in various forms, including juice, gel, and capsules.

15. Chamomile Powder

Chamomile, a flower from the daisy family, is known for its calming properties and use in digestive problems such as bloating, gas, and indigestion.

Scientific evidence

Limited research is available on chamomile's effectiveness in treating IBS. However, its antispasmodic and anti-inflammatory properties may relieve some IBS symptoms. Further research is needed to establish a direct connection.

How to use chamomile powder

Chamomile powder can be added to hot water to make tea. Follow the package instructions for the appropriate dosage.

16. Valerian Extract

Valerian, a perennial herb, is commonly used to help relieve anxiety, stress, and sleep disturbances. Its potential calming effects on the nervous system may help alleviate some IBS symptoms.

Scientific evidence

Although research on valerian extract's effectiveness for IBS is limited, its anti-anxiety and antispasmodic properties may relieve stress-related IBS symptoms. Further studies are needed to confirm these findings.

How to use valerian extract

Valerian extract is typically available as capsules, tablets, or tinctures.

17. Rosemary Extract

Rosemary, an evergreen shrub, has been used to treat digestive issues, including indigestion and bloating.

Scientific evidence

Limited research exists on rosemary extract's effectiveness for IBS. However, its antispasmodic and anti-inflammatory properties may provide some relief. More studies are needed to confirm these findings.

How to use rosemary extract

Rosemary extract is typically available as capsules, tablets, or liquid extracts.

18. Turmeric

Turmeric, a popular spice, contains curcumin, a compound known for its anti-inflammatory and antioxidant properties. It has been used to treat various gastrointestinal issues, including IBS.

Scientific evidence

Some studies suggest that turmeric may help improve IBS symptoms, such as abdominal pain and bloating. However, more research is needed to confirm these findings and establish the appropriate dosage.

How to use turmeric

Turmeric supplements are available in various forms, including capsules, tablets, and powders.

19. Melatonin

Melatonin is a sleep-promoting hormone produced in the pineal gland. However, it may also play a role in managing IBS symptoms. Melatonin is found in the digestive system at higher levels than in the blood or the pineal gland. This suggests that melatonin might play a significant role in helping the digestive system function properly.

Scientific evidence

In a 2005 study, researchers studied if melatonin 3 mg could help improve bowel symptoms and sleep issues in people with IBS who had trouble sleeping. After two weeks of taking melatonin, participants experienced a significant decrease in abdominal pain, but the treatment didn't affect other IBS symptoms or sleep quality. Another study published in 2023 investigated the effects of melatonin 3 mg twice a day on IBS symptoms, quality of life, and sleep in patients with and without sleep disorders. At the end of an 8-week trial period, results showed significant improvements in IBS symptoms and quality of life for both groups, and improved sleep parameters for those with sleep disorders. This suggests that melatonin could be an effective treatment for IBS patients, regardless of whether they have sleep issues.

How to use Melatonin

Melatonin is typically available as capsules, tablets, or liquid supplements. It is important to follow the recommended dosage provided by the manufacturer or as advised by a healthcare professional. Start with a low dose and gradually increase it as needed, ensuring not to exceed the recommended amount.

20. Ayurveda

Ayurveda, a 5,000-year-old traditional Indian medicine system, focuses on achieving balance in the body, mind, and spirit to maintain health. The word "Ayurveda" comes from two Sanskrit words: "ayur," meaning life, and "veda," meaning knowledge or science, so it is often referred to as the "science of life." Based on three fundamental energies (doshas), Ayurvedic treatments restore balance using natural remedies, dietary changes, and lifestyle modifications.

The history of Ayurveda dates back to ancient India, where it was developed by sages and practitioners who gained knowledge through meditation, observation, and experimentation. Ancient Ayurvedic texts, like the Charaka Samhita and the Sushruta Samhita, form the basis of this system of medicine.

Not many studies show that Ayurveda works for IBS, but there's one from 2023 that looked into it. They compared a traditional Ayurvedic remedy (Kalingadi Churna) to a "whole Ayurveda" approach to treating IBS. The study had 48 patients and lasted 60 days, studying symptom severity, relief, anxiety, depression, and quality of life. The "whole Ayurveda" approach made a more significant difference in IBS symptoms than just using Kalingadi Churna. But they didn't compare these treatments to a placebo, so there is still more to learn.

21. Homeopathy

Homeopathy has been in existence for over two centuries. It was created by a German doctor named Samuel Hahnemann. The core principle of homeopathy is "like cures like." This means that substances that cause symptoms in healthy people can potentially help treat someone with similar symptoms when prepared in a specific way.

To make homeopathic remedies, natural substances like plants or minerals are diluted in water or alcohol and then shaken. Interestingly, the more diluted and shaken the remedy, the stronger it is believed to be. This is different from traditional medicine, where higher concentrations usually mean more potent effects.

Homeopathy is used to address a wide variety of health issues, ranging from allergies to digestive problems. A homeopath will evaluate your symptoms, lifestyle, and overall health before selecting a customized remedy just for you. This usually comes in the form of tiny pellets that dissolve under your tongue.

Scientific evidence

The scientific validity of homeopathy is still a matter of debate. While many studies have been conducted, their results have been inconsistent. Some people believe that any positive effects are simply due to the placebo effect.

In 2013, a review was conducted on three studies that examined the use of homeopathy in treating IBS. However, the evidence provided was not significant due to some issues with the studies, such as short-term follow-ups and limited data. The review did suggest a possible benefit for a remedy called asafoetida for IBS-C, but it is important to approach the results with caution. Further high-quality research is needed to determine whether homeopathy is effective in treating IBS, especially in comparison to a placebo or usual care.

22. Moxibustion

Moxibustion is a traditional Chinese medicine (TCM) technique that involves burning a small, spongy herb called mugwort (Artemisia vulgaris) near specific acupuncture points on the body. Moxibustion warms these points, stimulates the flow of vital energy (Qi), and promotes blood circulation, which is believed to help with various health conditions, including IBS.

There are two main types:

1. **Direct moxibustion:** A small cone of dried mugwort is placed directly on an acupuncture point and burned. The cone is removed before it reaches the skin to avoid burns. This method can be further classified as scarring or non-scarring, depending on whether it leaves a scar on the skin.

2. **Indirect moxibustion:** Without direct contact, the practitioner holds a lit moxa stick (a cigar-shaped roll of dried mugwort) near the skin above the acupuncture point. The heat is applied until the patient feels a comfortable, warm sensation.

In the context of IBS, moxibustion is believed to help by:

- **Regulating the gastrointestinal (GI) system:** Moxibustion is thought to improve the movement and function of the GI tract, which may help alleviate IBS symptoms such as abdominal pain, bloating, and irregular bowel movements.
- **Reducing inflammation:** Moxibustion may have anti-inflammatory effects, which could help decrease inflammation in the gut and relieve IBS symptoms.
- **Balancing the autonomic nervous system:** The technique is believed to help regulate the balance between the sympathetic and parasympathetic nervous systems, which may positively impact IBS symptoms by reducing stress and promoting relaxation.
- **Strengthening the immune system:** Moxibustion may help boost the immune system, potentially reducing the risk of infections or other complications related to IBS.

Scientific evidence

While some studies suggest that moxibustion may benefit IBS patients, the evidence is still limited and of varying quality. More high-quality, large-scale clinical trials are needed to establish the effectiveness and safety of moxibustion as a treatment for IBS.

It is important to note that while these complementary and alternative treatments show potential in managing IBS symptoms, more research is needed to confirm their effectiveness and safety. Remember that these therapies should be used alongside conventional treatments and not as a replacement. These treatments may have a complementary role in treating IBS, especially in combination with other more proven therapies like diet, psychotherapies, and medications. Always consult your healthcare provider before starting any new treatment. They can help you determine the best course of action based on your individual needs and circumstances.

CHAPTER 10

The Battle with Bloating

"Sometimes the smallest step in the right direction ends up being the biggest step of your life. Tiptoe if you must but take the step."
- Naeem Callaway

Ah, bloating. That pesky, uncomfortable feeling that makes us feel like we've got a fully inflated balloon in our stomach. It is a common symptom of IBS, but various other factors can also cause it.

Bloating and belly swelling (also known as distention in medical terminology) are two of the most common tummy troubles people complain about when they come to see me at my clinic. In the US, surveys show that around 16% to 31% of people experience bloating from time to time. Almost everyone has felt a bit bloated or puffed up after a meal, right?

We can all agree that bloating is a nuisance, but what exactly is it? Bloating is the sensation of abdominal fullness, often accompanied by gas, discomfort, and sometimes pain. It can make our clothes feel tight, and let's be honest, it's not exactly a confidence booster. But it's essential to remember that bloating is a symptom, not a disease in itself.

Bloating can really mess with your quality of life and send you running to the doctor. But here's the thing: these symptoms are tricky to deal with. Figuring out the cause of bloating can be like solving a puzzle because so many different pieces can fit together.

And since bloating and belly swelling can be a bit vague, it can be challenging for healthcare professionals to figure out what's happening. In addition, bloating is often linked to gut-brain issues, which can be tough to treat.

In this chapter, I will try to help explain why we get bloated and how we manage it by giving you a practical guide on handling bloating and belly swelling. We'll discuss common reasons (as long as you don't have any red-flag symptoms (*See Chapter 4*). By looking at these possible causes, you can work with your healthcare provider to figure out the best way to tackle your bloating and belly swelling based on your unique situation.

Causes of bloating: it is not just IBS!

While IBS is a common cause of bloating, it's not the only one. Other potential culprits include:

- Diet: Certain foods, such as those high in fiber, fat, dairy (milk products), or FODMAPs, may contribute to the development of bloating.
- Stress: Stress and anxiety can exacerbate bloating in some patients.
- Certain medications: For example, non-steroidal anti-inflammatory drugs (NSAIDs), can cause bloating.
- Swallowing air: Eating too quickly, chewing gum, or drinking carbonated beverages can introduce excess air into the stomach.
- Constipation: When things slow down in the digestive tract, gas can build up, leading to bloating.

- Gastrointestinal disorders: Celiac disease, inflammatory bowel disease, and gastroparesis (slow stomach digestion) can cause bloating.
- Hormonal changes: Some women may experience bloating and water retention during their menstrual cycle.
- Small intestinal bacterial overgrowth (SIBO). *See Chapter 4 for more details.*
- Issues with the muscles that control your pelvic floor
- Physical blockage in the gut
- Chronic intestinal pseudo-obstruction (A condition that causes gut muscles not to work properly)
- Not enough digestive enzymes from the pancreas
- Low thyroid hormone levels (hypothyroidism)
- Fluid buildup in the belly (ascites)
- Fat collecting around the waist (central adiposity)
- Past stomach or esophagus surgery (like weight loss surgery or acid reflux surgery)
- Cancer in the gut or female reproductive system
- A weird thing called abdomino-phrenic dyssynergia. Let me explain what that means.

Abdomino-phrenic dyssynergia

Some people with belly swelling have too much gas inside their stomach, so their body responds in a strange way called abdomino-phrenic dyssynergia. Instead of the usual response where the belly muscles tighten, and the diaphragm (a muscle under the lungs) relaxes to make more space, the opposite happens. Researchers found that people with IBS, even if they didn't have a lot of gas inside, had their diaphragm tighten and move down while the belly muscles relax. This can make the belly stick out more than it should.

149

The science behind bloating

Bloating occurs when gas or air builds up in the gastrointestinal tract, causing the abdomen to expand. Bacteria in the colon can produce gas as they break down food, or it can be swallowed while eating or drinking. IBS sufferers often have an increased sensitivity to pain and sensations in the gut. This means that even average amounts of gas can cause feelings of bloating and discomfort.

Bloating be gone: treatment options

1. **Dietary modifications:** Patients with IBS with bloating may benefit from dietary modifications, such as reducing lactose/dairy, avoiding raw vegetables, reducing the intake of gas-producing foods (e.g., beans, lentils, broccoli, cabbage) and FODMAPs. Keep a food diary to identify and eliminate trigger foods.
2. **Probiotics:** These beneficial bacteria may help restore balance to the gut microbiome, reducing gas production and bloating. Some studies have shown that certain probiotics can improve bloating and other IBS symptoms. However, the efficacy of probiotics varies depending on the strain and dose used.
3. **Medications:** Antibiotics, such as rifaximin, can reduce bacterial overgrowth in the small intestine and improve bloating and other IBS symptoms. Other antibiotics used to treat SIBO, like Doxycycline, Metronidazole, etc., may help relieve bloating.
4. **Exercise:** Physical activity can help improve digestion and relieve constipation.
5. **Over-the-counter remedies:** Gas-relief medications like simethicone or activated charcoal can help break up gas bubbles in the stomach.

6. **Alternative therapies:** Acupuncture, yoga, and herbal remedies may offer relief for some people. Certain herbal remedies, such as peppermint or caraway oil, ginger, and chamomile, may help improve bloating in some patients.

7. **Mind-body techniques:** Stress can exacerbate bloating, so try relaxation techniques such as meditation, deep breathing, or progressive muscle relaxation.

8. **Biofeedback:** A technique that helps people learn to control their body's functions by monitoring and receiving feedback on physiological signals, such as heart rate or muscle tension. By becoming aware of these signals, individuals can make conscious adjustments to improve their physical or mental well-being.

At present, there is no test to diagnose abdomino-phrenic dyssynergia. However, studies have revealed that biofeedback treatment is an effective solution. In one study, 26 individuals experiencing gut problems and bloating underwent biofeedback therapy. This treatment involved a unique technique that demonstrated to the patients how their muscles functioned. As a result, they experienced a reduction in belly size, their diaphragm moved up, and they felt less bloated.

In another study, 44 patients with various gut issues and bloating after meals reported improvements following biofeedback therapy. Their chest muscles relaxed, their belly muscles functioned better, and they felt less bloated. If biofeedback therapy is not accessible, diaphragmatic breathing is a viable alternative. This simple technique has aided individuals with conditions such as rumination syndrome, excessive air swallowing, and belching. Although it has not been studied explicitly for bloating, it could serve a similar purpose to biofeedback by correcting how the body responds to it.

9. **Diaphragmatic breathing**

Diaphragmatic or belly breathing is a simple relaxation technique that helps you breathe more deeply and efficiently. It involves using your diaphragm, a large muscle located just below your lungs, to breathe air rather than relying on your chest and shoulders.

Here's how to practice diaphragmatic breathing:

- **Find a comfortable position:** You can sit or lie down, whatever feels best for you. Make sure your body is relaxed, and your head, neck, and shoulders are supported.
- **Place one hand on your chest and the other on your abdomen:** This will help you monitor your breathing and ensure you are using your diaphragm correctly.
- **Inhale slowly through your nose:** As you breathe, let your belly expand and fill with air while keeping your chest still. You should feel the hand on your abdomen rise.
- **Exhale slowly through your mouth:** As you breathe out, let your belly deflate and feel the hand on your abdomen lower. You can gently press on your abdomen to help release the air.
- **Repeat and focus on your breath:** Continue to practice slow, deep breaths, focusing on the sensation of your breath moving in and out. Aim for about five to ten minutes a day or whenever you feel stressed.

Diaphragmatic breathing can also help you relax, reduce stress, and improve overall well-being. Practice regularly to make it a natural part of your daily routine.

The following flow chart will give you a good idea of managing your bloating and gas.

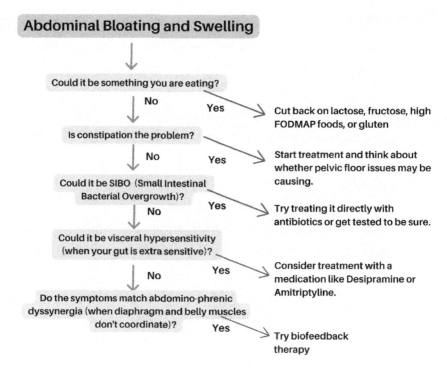

Adapted with permission from Cangemi DJ, et al. A Practical Approach to the Diagnosis and Treatment of Abdominal Bloating and Distension. Gastroenterol Hepatol (N Y). 2022 Feb;18(2):75-84.

In conclusion, bloating may be a common and uncomfortable symptom, but it doesn't have to rule your life. By understanding its causes, seeking appropriate treatments, and practicing self-care, you can have relief and regain control of your life. Remember, you're not alone in this battle; plenty of resources and support are available to help you along the way. So, keep your chin up, and let's kick bloating to the curb!

Key takeaways:

- Bloating is a common symptom of IBS, but various other factors can cause it.
- Figuring out the cause of bloating can be like solving a puzzle because so many pieces can fit together.
- Bloating is often linked to gut-brain issues, which can be tough to treat.
- Bloating is a symptom, not a disease in itself.
- Possible causes of bloating include diet, stress, certain medications, swallowing air, constipation, gastrointestinal disorders, hormonal changes, SIBO, pelvic floor problems, physical blockage in the gut, and more.
- Bloating occurs when gas or air builds up in the gastrointestinal tract, causing the abdomen to expand.
- Treatment options for bloating include dietary modifications, probiotics, medications, exercise, over-the-counter remedies, alternative therapies, mind-body techniques, biofeedback, and diaphragmatic breathing.
- Diaphragmatic breathing, also known as belly breathing, is a simple relaxation technique that can help with bloating and improve overall well-being.
- The flow chart provided in the chapter can help manage bloating and gas.
- By understanding the causes of bloating, seeking appropriate treatments, and practicing self-care, relief can be achieved, and control of life can be regained.

CHAPTER 11

Women and IBS: Unique Challenges and Connections

"Here's to strong women: May we know them, may we be them, may we raise them." - Unknown

---

Women experience IBS differently than men, and several unique factors contribute to their symptoms. It has been found in some studies that women with IBS have a higher chance of getting unnecessary surgeries, like hysterectomies or ovarian surgeries. This may be due to doctors mistakenly attributing their abdominal pain symptoms to gynecological causes. But at the same time, in carefully selected patients with chronic pelvic pain, 74% and 95% of women will report complete or significant pain relief following a hysterectomy.

This chapter will explore the connections between IBS and women's health, including sexual function, chronic pelvic pain, endometriosis, menstrual cycles, pregnancy, and menopause.

Sexual function

Sexual dysfunction, like a lower sex drive or painful intercourse, is more common in people with IBS. A recent study in Poland showed that as many as 48% of female IBS patients attending an outpatient clinic experienced sexual dysfunction. The severity of sexual dysfunction is related to the intensity of IBS symptoms.

There could be several reasons for this observation. One significant factor is visceral hypersensitivity, which plays a crucial role in IBS. The bowel expansion due to gas or fluid can be uncomfortable or even painful. This sensitivity may be unique to visceral organs, such as the digestive system, glands, and vagina, rather than a general increase in pain sensitivity.

Chronic Pelvic Pain

Chronic pelvic pain (CPP) is common in women, affecting around 15-24% of females worldwide. It is defined as pain in the pelvic region lasting six months or more, and its causes can be complex and varied. Considerable overlap exists between CPP and IBS. Research indicates that as many as 50% of women with CPP also suffer from IBS, while at least 30% of women with IBS experience chronic pelvic pain.

The exact reason for the overlap between CPP and IBS is unclear. Researchers suggest that a combination of factors may play a role in causing the condition, such as increased sensitivity to sensations in the gut, changes in the movement of food through the digestive system, and heightened sensitivity to pain in the nervous system.

The treatment for CPP and IBS often involves a multidisciplinary approach, including medications for pain relief, physical therapy, and psychological interventions, such as cognitive-behavioral therapy. Addressing the underlying causes of both CPP and IBS can lead to better symptom management and improved quality of life for women affected by these conditions.

Endometriosis and IBS

Endometriosis is a gynecological condition that affects approximately 10% of reproductive-aged women. It occurs when endometrial tissue, which typically lines the uterus, grows outside the uterus, leading to inflammation, pain, and, in some cases, infertility. Research has shown that women with endometriosis are more likely to experience IBS symptoms. One study reported a 3.5 times higher risk of having IBS in women with endometriosis.

The relationship between endometriosis and IBS is complex and not fully understood. Some researchers suggest that endometriosis-associated inflammation could lead to changes in the gastrointestinal tract, contributing to IBS symptoms. Additionally, shared risk factors, such as hormonal fluctuations and genetic predisposition, may explain why these conditions can occur together.

Treatment for women with both endometriosis and IBS often involves addressing the underlying endometriosis. The treatment may involve hormonal therapies, pain medications, surgery, and managing IBS symptoms through dietary modifications, medications, and stress reduction techniques.

Menstrual cycle

Hormonal fluctuations during the menstrual cycle can exacerbate IBS symptoms in women. IBS symptoms, such as abdominal pain and bloating, are more severe in the premenstrual and menstrual phases. This may be due to increased progesterone levels and decreased estrogen levels during these phases, which can affect gut motility and sensitivity.

Menopause

Menopause, the natural biological process marking the end of a woman's menstrual cycle, can also influence IBS symptoms. Studies show that women often see an improvement in their IBS symptoms after they go through menopause. However, many women also notice that their IBS symptoms get worse when they are just starting to enter menopause, a phase called perimenopause.

Some experts believe that this increase in symptoms around menopause time might be linked to a drop in sex hormones, like how IBS symptoms can get worse around the start of a woman's period. The exact relationship between menopause and IBS is poorly understood, but hormonal changes may play a role. Hormone replacement therapy (HRT) has been shown to improve IBS symptoms in some women, but more research is needed to determine its effectiveness.

IBS and pregnancy: a delicate balance

Pregnancy is an amazing adventure, but it can feel like a bumpy ride for women with IBS. It is important to note that every woman's IBS and pregnancy journey is different. Some women might find relief from symptoms like abdominal pain, bloating, constipation, or diarrhea. In contrast, others may experience a worsening condition or no change.

Fluctuations occur due to hormonal shifts during pregnancy, particularly a rise in progesterone levels. This hormone is essential for maintaining the pregnancy and relaxing the uterine muscles, but it can also affect the digestive system, resulting in alterations in bowel movements.

Higher progesterone levels can slow down digestion, causing constipation for some women. For others, the hormonal changes may make their GI tract more sensitive or overactive, leading to diarrhea or increased abdominal pain.

Handling IBS during pregnancy requires a customized approach. Some treatments for non-pregnant women might not be suitable for expectant mothers.

Here are a few management strategies for pregnant women with IBS:

- **Diet:** Emphasize a balanced, nutritious diet for your and your baby's health. Pregnant women with IBS may need to adjust their diets, like increasing fiber intake for constipation or trying a low-FODMAP diet for gas and bloating.
- **Exercise:** Participate in gentle, low-impact exercises like walking, swimming, or prenatal yoga to alleviate stress, encourage regular bowel movements, and improve overall well-being. Consult your healthcare provider before starting any exercise program during pregnancy.
- **Stress management:** Since stress can worsen IBS symptoms, practicing relaxation techniques during pregnancy is vital. Consider deep breathing exercises, mindfulness meditation, or prenatal yoga to help manage stress levels.
- **Prenatal care:** Regular prenatal care is crucial for all pregnant women, including those with IBS. Keep your obstetrician informed about your IBS symptoms and any changes you experience during pregnancy. They can help monitor your condition and provide guidance for managing your IBS while ensuring a healthy pregnancy.
- **Medication:** Some IBS medications might not be safe during pregnancy. Consult your healthcare provider before taking any medication, including over-the-counter treatments, while

pregnant. They can suggest safe alternatives to manage your IBS symptoms during pregnancy.

IBS medications considered generally safe during pregnancy:

Fiber supplements: Psyllium (Metamucil), calcium polycarbophil (FiberCon), methylcellulose (Citrucel).

Laxatives: Over-the-counter options like MiraLAX can be used short-term for constipation relief.

Antispasmodics: Some antispasmodic medications like dicyclomine (Bentyl) may be used.

Medications to be avoided or used with caution during pregnancy:

Antidepressants: Tricyclic antidepressants like amitriptyline (Elavil) and SSRIs like fluoxetine (Prozac) should be used cautiously, as their safety during pregnancy is not well-established.

Linaclotide (Linzess), Lubiprostone (Amitiza), and Plecanatide (Trulance): These medications are classified as Pregnancy Category C, meaning that there is not enough information about their safety during pregnancy. Use them only if the potential benefits outweigh the potential risks. The risk of fetal harm is less likely as these medications have minimal absorption into the bloodstream.

Alosetron (Lotronex): This medication is not recommended during pregnancy due to limited safety data.

Eluxadoline (Viberzi): There is limited information on its safety during pregnancy, so it should be used cautiously. No known risk has been reported in animal studies.

Rifaximin (Xifaxan): This medication is classified as Pregnancy Category C. It should be used only if the potential benefits outweigh the potential risks. The risk of fetal harm is not expected as this medication has minimal absorption into the bloodstream. Avoid during 1st trimester.

Opioid-based medications: These medications, such as loperamide (Imodium), should be used with caution during pregnancy and only under the supervision of a healthcare provider.

Women with IBS face unique challenges due to the interplay of hormones, reproductive health, and other women-specific conditions. Understanding the connections between IBS and conditions like sexual health, chronic pelvic pain, endometriosis, menstrual cycles, pregnancy, and menopause, can help healthcare providers develop personalized treatment plans for their female patients.

Collaborating with a healthcare team, including gastroenterologists, gynecologists, obstetricians, and dietitians, can help women with IBS navigate the complexities of their condition and improve their overall quality of life.

Key takeaways:

- Women with IBS have unique symptoms compared to men. They may be at risk of unnecessary surgeries due to misdiagnosis of gynecological causes for abdominal pain.
- Sexual dysfunction is more common in women with IBS and may be related to visceral hypersensitivity.
- Chronic pelvic pain and IBS have a high overlap, possibly due to factors such as altered gut motility and central sensitization.

- Due to shared risk factors, women with endometriosis are more likely to experience IBS symptoms. Inflammation may contribute to the co-occurrence of these conditions.
- Hormonal fluctuations during the menstrual cycle and menopause can exacerbate IBS symptoms, and treatment may involve hormone replacement therapy.
- Pregnancy can affect IBS symptoms. The management strategies for pregnant women with IBS include dietary adjustments, exercise, stress management, regular prenatal care, and careful medication selection.
- Collaborating with a healthcare team can help women with IBS navigate the complexities of their condition and improve their overall quality of life.

CHAPTER 12

Managing and Coping with IBS

"Believe you can, and you're halfway there." - Theodore Roosevelt

Lifestyle changes for managing IBS symptoms

Strategies for self-care

Living with IBS can be challenging, but prioritizing self-care and managing stress can improve your quality of life and better cope with your symptoms. We will explore self-care strategies and stress management techniques to empower and encourage those with IBS.

The Importance of self-care for IBS

Self-care is essential for everyone but especially crucial for those with IBS. By taking care of your physical, emotional, and mental well-being, you can better manage your symptoms and reduce the impact of IBS on your daily life. Investing in self-care can lead to increased resilience, improved mood, and a greater sense of control over your condition.

Creating a self-care routine

A self-care routine is a personalized plan that outlines the activities and practices you will engage in to maintain your overall well-being. Consider incorporating the following elements into your routine:

- **Regular exercise:** Physical activity can help reduce stress, improve mood, and promote better digestion. Aim for at least 30 minutes of moderate exercise at least 3 days a week.
- **Balanced diet:** A nutritious and balanced diet can help manage IBS symptoms. Work with a healthcare professional or dietitian to develop a personalized meal plan that considers your triggers and preferences.
- **Sleep hygiene:** Prioritize getting enough quality sleep by establishing a consistent sleep schedule, creating a relaxing bedtime routine, and making your sleep environment comfortable.
- **Mindfulness and relaxation techniques:** Practices like meditation, deep breathing exercises, and progressive muscle relaxation can help reduce stress and promote a sense of calm.
- **Social connections:** Foster strong relationships with friends and family who can provide emotional support and understanding.
- **Hobbies and interests:** Engage in activities that bring you joy and help you relax, such as reading, gardening, or painting.

Setting boundaries and prioritizing self-care

Setting boundaries and prioritizing self-care are essential. Communicate your needs with your friends, family, and coworkers. Don't be afraid to ask for help or accommodations when necessary. Remember that taking care of yourself is not selfish; it's a vital aspect of managing your IBS and maintaining your overall well-being.

Exercise and physical activity for IBS

As discussed earlier, regular exercise and physical activity can have numerous benefits for people with IBS. Some of the advantages include the following:

- **Stress reduction:** Physical activity can help reduce stress, which exacerbates IBS symptoms.
- **Enhanced mood:** Exercise releases endorphins, which can help improve mood and alleviate anxiety and depression often associated with IBS.
- **Increased energy levels:** Regular physical activity can increase energy and overall well-being.
- **Improved digestion:** Exercise promotes regular bowel movements and can help alleviate constipation, a common symptom of IBS.

Choosing the proper exercise for you

When it comes to exercise and physical activity, choosing activities you enjoy and can maintain in the long term is essential. Some options to consider include the following:

- **Aerobic exercises:** Walking, swimming, cycling, and dancing are low-impact aerobic exercises that can help improve cardiovascular health and digestion.
- **Strength training:** Incorporating resistance training, such as weightlifting or bodyweight exercises, can help build muscle, increase metabolism, and improve overall fitness.
- **Flexibility exercises:** Practicing yoga, Pilates, or stretching can help improve flexibility, reduce stress, and promote relaxation.

Sleep hygiene and IBS

Proper sleep hygiene is crucial for managing IBS symptoms and maintaining overall well-being. Poor sleep can increase stress and fatigue and worsen IBS symptoms. Here are some tips for improving your sleep hygiene:

- **Establish a regular sleep schedule:** Go to bed and wake up at the same time every day, even on weekends, to help regulate your body's internal clock.
- **Create a relaxing bedtime routine:** Engage in calming activities before bedtime, such as reading a book, taking a warm bath, or practicing relaxation techniques.
- **Optimize your sleep environment:** Ensure your bedroom is dark, quiet, and comfortable. Use blackout curtains, a white noise machine, or earplugs to block disruptions.
- **Limit exposure to screens before bed:** The blue light emitted by smartphones, tablets, and computers can interfere with your body's production of melatonin, a hormone that promotes sleep. Aim to stop using screens at least an hour before bedtime.
- **Watch your diet:** Be mindful of what you eat and drink in the hours leading up to bedtime. Avoid consuming large meals, caffeine, or alcohol close to bedtime, as they can disrupt sleep.

By incorporating these lifestyle modifications, individuals with IBS can manage their symptoms and improve their quality of life. However, remember that each person's experience with IBS is unique. What works for one person may not work for another. So, come up with your own routine with diet, exercise, relaxation, and sleep that suits your body.

IBS in Special Populations

IBS can affect anyone, but it can affect certain populations differently. Let's talk about IBS in special populations, such as children, the elderly, pregnant women, and men and women in general.

IBS in children

IBS is common in children, and approximately 14% of children experience IBS symptoms at some point during childhood. These symptoms, such as abdominal pain, diarrhea, and constipation, can negatively impact their quality of life and social functioning. However, IBS in children is often not diagnosed or treated correctly.

For children, management and coping strategies include creating a structured routine with regular meals, naps, and playtime. Children thrive on consistency, so having a predictable daily routine can help them feel safe and secure. Additionally, parents can teach their children coping skills such as deep breathing exercises, visualization, and positive self-talk. It's also important to communicate openly with children and validate their emotions, helping them to feel heard and understood.

Talking to a healthcare provider is essential if your child has IBS symptoms. Treatment options may include changes to their diet, stress management techniques, or medications like fiber supplements or laxatives. Encouraging regular exercise and good sleep habits can also help.

For more information on IBS in children and adolescents, visit https://aboutkidsgi.org/.

IBS in the elderly

People may be more likely to develop IBS as they age due to changes in gut motility, gut microbiome, and underlying medical conditions. Unfortunately, IBS in the elderly is often underdiagnosed and under-treated due to the perception that it's only a "young person's disease." Elderly individuals with IBS may also have additional challenges like mobility issues and medication interactions.

The elderly may face physical limitations that impact their daily activities, making managing and coping with these limitations important. Regular exercise, a balanced diet, and staying socially connected can help improve overall physical and mental health. Caregivers can also provide support and assistance with daily activities to help seniors maintain their independence as much as possible. Coping strategies for older adults can include practicing mindfulness, engaging in hobbies, and seeking support from friends, family, or support groups.

If you are an elderly individual experiencing IBS symptoms, speaking with a healthcare provider is important. Treatment options may include changes to your diet, stress management techniques, and medications like laxatives or antispasmodics. Additionally, it is essential to address any other medical conditions or medications that may contribute to IBS symptoms.

IBS during pregnancy

IBS symptoms can worsen or improve during pregnancy, and it is estimated that 30-50% of pregnant women experience gastrointestinal symptoms like constipation, diarrhea, and abdominal pain. Pregnant women with IBS may face other challenges like nausea, vomiting, and food aversions. Seek medical advice from a healthcare provider before taking any medication or making significant changes to your diet or lifestyle during pregnancy.

Tips for managing IBS during pregnancy:

- **Eat small, frequent meals:** Eating smaller meals throughout the day can help reduce bloating and discomfort associated with IBS. It can also help prevent nausea and vomiting, which are common during pregnancy.
- **Avoid trigger foods:** Avoid foods that trigger your IBS symptoms. Common triggers include high-fat foods, caffeine, spicy foods, and carbonated drinks.
- **Stay hydrated:** Drink plenty of water to keep yourself hydrated. Dehydration can worsen constipation, a common symptom of IBS during pregnancy.
- **Exercise:** Gentle exercises, such as walking or yoga, can help alleviate constipation and reduce stress, which can worsen IBS symptoms.
- **Practice stress management techniques:** Pregnancy can be a stressful time, so it is important to practice stress management techniques like deep breathing, meditation, or yoga to help reduce stress and manage IBS symptoms.

For more information on IBS during pregnancy, please visit:

International Foundation for Gastrointestinal Disorders. IBS during Pregnancy. Available at https://aboutibs.org/what-is-ibs/ibs-in-women/

Coping strategies for living with IBS

Relaxation Techniques

Stress can exacerbate IBS symptoms, so developing effective stress management strategies is essential. Here are some techniques to consider:

- **Deep breathing exercises:** Deep breathing exercises can help reduce stress and promote relaxation. To practice deep breathing, find a quiet and comfortable place to sit. Take a deep breath through your nose and hold it for a few seconds, then exhale slowly through your mouth.
- **Progressive muscle relaxation:** Progressive muscle relaxation involves tensing and relaxing different muscle groups to promote relaxation. To practice progressive muscle relaxation, find a quiet, comfortable place to lie down. Tense your muscles in one part of your body, such as your arms, and hold for a few seconds before relaxing.
- **Mindfulness meditation:** Mindfulness meditation involves focusing on the present moment and accepting thoughts and feelings without judgment. To practice mindfulness meditation, find a quiet and comfortable place to sit. Focus on your breath and bring your attention to the present moment.
- **Visualization or guided imagery:** This technique involves using your imagination to create calming, peaceful images in your mind, helping to reduce stress and promote a sense of calm.
- **Mind-body exercises:** Activities like tai chi and qigong combine gentle physical movements with deep breathing and mindfulness to help reduce stress and improve overall well-being.

- **Support groups:** Connecting with others with similar experiences and challenges can provide emotional support, understanding, and practical advice for managing IBS-related stress.
- **Consider therapy or counseling:** A mental health professional can guide you on coping strategies and help address any emotional challenges related to IBS.

Strategies for managing emotional symptoms

To better cope with the emotional challenges of IBS, consider incorporating the following strategies:

- **Journaling:** Writing about your thoughts and feelings can provide an outlet for emotions and help you gain insight into your experiences.
- **Physical activity:** Regular exercise can help reduce stress, improve mood, and promote better digestion.
- **Social support:** Connecting with friends, family, and others who understand your experiences can provide emotional support and practical advice.
- **Time management:** Establishing a daily routine and prioritizing tasks can help you feel more in control and reduce stress.

Benefits of therapy and support groups

Seeking professional help, such as therapy or support groups, can provide invaluable guidance and encouragement in managing the emotional challenges of IBS. Therapists can offer coping strategies and support, while support groups provide a safe space to connect with others who share similar experiences. *See Chapter 10 for more details.*

Advocating for yourself and others with IBS

- **Educate yourself:** Stay informed about the latest IBS research, treatment options, and resources. This will empower you to make informed decisions about your care and advocate for your needs.
- **Speak up:** Share your experiences and advocate for your needs with friends, family, and healthcare providers.
- **Share your story:** Connect with others with IBS through support groups, online forums, or social media. Sharing your experiences can encourage and support others, helping you feel understood and less isolated.
- **Raise awareness:** Use your voice to educate others about IBS and promote understanding and compassion for those living with the condition. Participate in awareness campaigns, events, and discussions to help break down misconceptions and stigma surrounding IBS.
- **Support others:** Connect with others living with IBS through support groups and social media, offering encouragement and sharing your insights.

The Importance of self-compassion and self-acceptance

- **Be kind to yourself:** Recognize that living with IBS can be daunting, and sometimes feeling frustrated or overwhelmed is okay.
- **Recognize your strengths:** Focus on your positive qualities and accomplishments rather than solely on your IBS symptoms and limitations.
- **Embrace your emotions:** Acknowledge and accept positive and negative feelings without judgment. This can help create a healthier relationship with yourself.

- **Practice self-compassion:** Treat yourself with the same understanding and empathy you would offer to a friend with a similar condition.
- **Acknowledge progress:** Celebrate small victories and recognize the steps you are taking to manage your IBS.

The emotional and psychological impact of IBS - building emotional resilience

Living with IBS can have significant emotional and psychological consequences, including feelings of embarrassment, isolation, and frustration. It is essential to recognize the impact IBS can have on your mental health and seek appropriate support and resources to help manage these challenges.

Developing emotional resilience can help you better cope with the ups and downs of living with IBS. Some strategies for building resilience include:

- **Cultivating a positive outlook:** Focus on your strengths and accomplishments and try to maintain a sense of hope and optimism.
- **Setting realistic goals:** Break larger tasks into smaller, achievable steps, and celebrate your progress along the way.
- **Developing problem-solving skills:** Learn to approach challenges with a proactive, solution-focused mindset.
- **Embracing self-care:** Prioritize taking care of your physical, emotional, and mental well-being to manage stress better and improve your overall quality of life.

Developing a personalized treatment plan

- **Work with your healthcare team:** Collaborate with your doctor, dietitian, and other healthcare professionals to create a tailored plan that addresses your unique needs.
- **Experiment and adapt:** Be open to trying new strategies and adjusting your treatment plan as needed.
- **Track your symptoms:** Maintain a food and symptom diary to identify potential triggers and patterns. This can help inform adjustments to your treatment plan.
- **Be patient and flexible:** Finding the right treatment plan may take time and require adjustments. Stay open to trying new approaches and communicate any changes in your symptoms to your healthcare team.
- **Monitor your progress:** Keep a symptom diary to track your triggers, dietary changes, and the effectiveness of treatments.

Practical tips for coping with symptoms of IBS:

1. **Identify your triggers:** Keep a food diary to track what you eat and how it affects your symptoms. This can help you identify trigger foods and avoid them in the future.
2. **Mindful eating:** Take your time while eating. Chew your food slowly and thoroughly. Eating in a relaxed atmosphere can help prevent symptoms.
3. **Manage stress:** Stress can trigger IBS symptoms. To reduce stress, practice relaxation techniques such as deep breathing, meditation, or yoga.
4. **Exercise regularly:** Regular exercise can help reduce stress and improve bowel function. Try to engage in some form of physical activity every day.

5. **Stay hydrated:** Drinking plenty of water can help prevent constipation and improve overall digestive function.

6. **Avoid alcohol and caffeine:** Alcohol and caffeine can irritate the gut and trigger IBS symptoms.

7. **Consider probiotics:** Probiotics are beneficial bacteria that help balance the gut microbiome and improve IBS symptoms.

8. **Try fiber supplements:** Fiber supplements such as psyllium or methylcellulose can help regulate bowel function and reduce constipation.

9. **Talk to your health care provider:** If your symptoms persist, talk to your doctor about medications or other treatments that may help.

With the right management strategies, living a full and active life with IBS is possible. Combining dietary changes, lifestyle modifications, and stress management techniques can help manage IBS symptoms.

CHAPTER 13

Finding Support for IBS

"You are never alone. You are eternally connected with everyone."
- Amit Ray

As a gastroenterologist who has dealt with IBS for many years, I strongly emphasize the importance of a support network. In this chapter, we will explore various ways to find support and connect with others who share similar experiences. We will also discuss how to talk to loved ones about IBS and find a healthcare provider who truly understands your condition.

Be an IBS champion

When you have IBS, you are not alone. By advocating for yourself and others, you can help improve understanding and management of this condition. Here are some simple ways to become an IBS champion:

1. **Share your story:** Share your IBS journey with friends, family, and colleagues to create awareness and help others feel comfortable discussing their experiences.
2. **Stay informed:** Keep up with the latest IBS research, treatments, and strategies, and share your insights with others to create a more understanding environment.

3. **Connect with the IBS community:** Join online forums, support groups, and social media communities to engage with fellow IBS warriors and contribute to a collective effort to improve lives.

4. **Partner with your healthcare team:** Communicate openly with your healthcare providers, ask questions, and provide feedback on your treatment plan for better outcomes.

5. **Get involved in local events:** Participate in IBS-related events like awareness walks, fundraisers, or educational workshops to raise funds and foster a sense of community.

6. **Support IBS organizations:** Volunteer your time, skills, or financial resources to help IBS organizations and research efforts.

7. **Encourage workplace accommodations:** Discuss your IBS with your employer and request reasonable accommodations to manage your symptoms at work.

By advocating for yourself and others with IBS, you're helping create a world where this condition is better understood and supported. Together, we can make a difference!

Online and in-person support groups for people with IBS

In today's digital age, finding support groups that cater to individuals with IBS is easier than ever. Online forums, social media platforms, and dedicated websites offer a safe space to share your experiences, seek advice, and learn from others.

Online forums

Websites like IBSgroup.org and the IBS Network offer discussion boards where you can ask questions, share tips, and connect with fellow IBS sufferers.

- **IBSgroup.org:** A comprehensive online forum allowing users to share their experiences, ask questions, and support one another. The forum is divided into categories based on different aspects of IBS, making finding the information you need easy. https://www.ibsgroup.org/forums/

- **The IBS Network:** A national charity in the UK that offers support and information to individuals with IBS. Their website provides many resources, including an online forum to connect with others experiencing similar challenges. https://www.theibsnetwork.org/

- **HealthBoards:** A popular online community focused on health-related topics. Their IBS board (www.healthboards.com/boards/irritable-bowel-syndrome-ibs) is dedicated to discussions about IBS symptoms, treatments, and coping strategies.

- **HealingWell:** An online community that focuses on chronic illness and health-related topics. The IBS forum (www.healingwell.com/community/default.aspx?f=26) is a space where people can share their experiences, ask questions, and seek support for dealing with IBS.

- **MedHelp:** A health-focused online community where people can ask questions and get answers from experts and peers. The IBS community (https://www.medhelp.org/forums/Irritable-Bowel-Syndrome-IBS/show/179) is dedicated to discussions about IBS symptoms, treatments, and living with the condition.

Social media groups

Facebook, Reddit, and other social platforms have numerous groups dedicated to IBS. Search for "IBS support group" or a similar term to find a community that suits your needs.

Facebook groups:

- IBS Support (closed group-may request access): https://www.facebook.com/groups/IBSsupport/
- Irritable Bowel Syndrome (IBS) support group (closed group-may request access): https://www.facebook.com/groups/Ibsprobs/
- Low FODMAP Diet for IBS (closed group-may request access): https://www.facebook.com/groups/139633278050276/

Twitter accounts:

- IBS Network (@IBSnetwork): https://twitter.com/IBSnetwork
- International Foundation for Gastrointestinal Disorders (@IFFGD): https://twitter.com/IFFGD
- Monash FODMAP (@MonashFODMAP): https://twitter.com/MonashFODMAP

Instagram accounts:

- The IBS Network (@theibsnetwork): https://www.instagram.com/theibsnetwork/
- Monash FODMAP (@monashfodmap): https://www.instagram.com/monashfodmap/

- The FODMAP Formula (@ fodmapformula): https://www.instagram.com/fodmapformula/

Reddit:

- **r/ibs**: A Reddit community dedicated to discussing IBS, where users can ask questions, share tips, and connect with others who understand their struggles. https://www.reddit.com/r/ibs/

Please note that the privacy settings of these groups may change over time, and some may require you to request membership before you can access their content. I always advise caution when sharing personal information online and remember that the advice shared in these groups should not replace the guidance of a qualified healthcare professional.

In-person support groups

Local hospitals, community centers, or organizations like the International Foundation for Gastrointestinal Disorders (IFFGD) may offer in-person support groups. Check their websites or call them to inquire about available options.

Digital apps for IBS: managing your symptoms with technology

Using smartphone digital apps can simplify symptom tracking, help you manage your diet, and promote a healthier lifestyle. This section will discuss using IBS apps and list ten popular options with a brief description, cost, and pros and cons for each app.

Download IBS apps from your device's app store (Apple App Store for iOS or Google Play Store for Android). Once installed, you'll typically need to create an account or sign in with an existing one. After that, you can explore symptom tracking, food diaries, and relaxation exercises. Here are ten popular IBS apps:

- **MySymptoms Food Diary** (iOS, Android): Track food intake, symptoms, and triggers.
  Cost: $2.99 (iOS), $3.49 (Android)
  Pros: Comprehensive tracking, personalized analysis
  Cons: No diet recommendations or support

- **Cara Care** (iOS, Android): Personalized guidance, symptom tracking, and gut health tips.
  Cost: Free, with in-app purchases for premium features
  Pros: Comprehensive, expert guidance
  Cons: Some premium features require payment

- **Bowelle** (iOS): Simple tracking of food, symptoms, bowel movements, and more.
  Cost: Free
  Pros: User-friendly, clear symptom overview
  Cons: iOS only, limited additional resources

- **Low FODMAP diet A to Z** (iOS, Android): Low FODMAP diet food identification.
  Cost: Free
  Pros: Each FODMAP rating is divided into categories, including oligosaccharides, fructose, polyols, and lactose content. You can effortlessly search for foods by their name and filter them by category or rating to find exactly what you need.
  Cons: Narrow focus on the low FODMAP diet

- **Monash University FODMAP Diet** (iOS, Android): Low FODMAP food guide, recipes, and symptom diary.
  Cost: $9.00 (iOS), $7.99 (Android)

Pros: Comprehensive low FODMAP resource, created by the diet's developers

Cons: Cost, limited to low FODMAP diet

- **Mahana** (iOS, Android): A 12-week CBT program for IBS management.

   Cost: No free trial. Costs $199/per 12-week program.

   Pros: IBS-specific focus, FDA-cleared, clinically validated, prescription digital therapeutic CBT.

   Cons: Expensive, limited to 12 weeks only.

- **Nerva: IBS Hypnotherapy** (iOS, Android): 6-week gut-directed hypnotherapy program.

   Cost: Free trial, $59.99 for full access

   Pros: Clinically backed approach, guided sessions

   Cons: Cost, limited to hypnotherapy

- **Zemedy** (iOS, Android): Cognitive Behavioral Therapy (CBT) app for IBS.

   Cost: Free trial, subscription pricing for full access

   Pros: CBT-based, personalized plans, supportive community

   Cons: Cost, limited to the CBT approach

- **FODMAP Helper** (Android): Low FODMAP diet companion, food diary, and meal planner.

   Cost: Free, with in-app purchases for premium features

   Pros: Large food database, meal planning

   Cons: Focus on the low FODMAP diet. Android only. Some features require payment

- **MyHealthyGut** (iOS): Gut health and nutrition app with meal plans, recipes, and symptom tracking.

   Cost: Free trial, subscription required for full access

   Pros: Comprehensive nutrition resources, gluten-free and low FODMAP support

Cons: Subscription cost, iOS only

By using these digital apps, you can better understand your IBS triggers, manage your symptoms, and maintain a healthier lifestyle. Each app offers unique features, so explore them to find the one that best fits your needs. Remember to discuss your IBS management plan with your healthcare provider to ensure you use the most effective strategies for your situation.

How to talk to loved ones about IBS

Talking to loved ones about IBS can be tricky, but it is crucial for building understanding and support. Here are some tips to help you have those conversations:

- **Choose the right time and place:** Select a calm, private setting for discussing your IBS to minimize distractions and allow for an open conversation.
- **Be honest and open:** Share your IBS experiences, symptoms, and triggers with your loved ones, so they can better understand your condition and support you.
- **Provide educational resources:** Offer articles, websites, or books to help your friends and family better understand IBS and its impact on your life.
- **Set boundaries:** Communicate your limitations and ask for understanding and support when you need to modify plans or opt out of certain activities due to your IBS symptoms.
- **Share your needs:** Let your loved ones know how they can support you, whether by offering a listening ear, helping with meal planning or simply being patient during flare-ups.
- **Keep the conversation ongoing:** Maintain open lines of communication with your loved ones, update them on your IBS

management journey, and discuss any new challenges or successes.

Tips for finding a healthcare provider who understands IBS

A knowledgeable and empathetic healthcare provider is crucial for effectively managing IBS. Here are some tips to help you find the right provider:

- **Ask** for recommendations from friends, family, or support groups
- **Research** potential providers online and check their credentials
- **Prepare** a list of questions to ask them to gauge their understanding of IBS
- **Trust** your instincts during your appointment and look for a provider who shows genuine concern for your well-being

Remember that finding support for IBS is essential to managing your condition and improving your quality of life. Advocate for yourself and others and connect with online or in-person support groups. Use apps to track symptoms and maintain a healthy lifestyle, emphasizing the importance of a support network for effectively managing IBS.

Key Takeaways:

- Be an IBS champion: Advocate for yourself and others to increase awareness and support.
- Online and in-person support groups: Connect with others via forums, social media, and local groups.

- Apps for IBS: Use technology to track symptoms, monitor diet, and maintain a healthier lifestyle.
- Talking to loved ones: Choose the right setting, be honest, explain IBS, and share your needs.
- Finding a healthcare provider: Seek recommendations, and research credentials, prepare questions, and trust your instincts.
- Emphasize the importance of a support network for effectively managing IBS and improving quality of life.

CHAPTER 14

Living a Full Life with IBS - Work, Travel, and Social Life

"Happiness is not something readymade. It comes from your own actions." - Dalai Lama XIV

This chapter will offer tips to help you navigate various aspects of life with IBS, including work, travel, and social situations.

Traveling with IBS

Traveling can be an exciting and enjoyable experience. Still, it may also have some unique challenges for those with IBS. With proper planning and some practical strategies, you can manage your IBS symptoms while on the go and make the most of your travels.

Tips for managing IBS symptoms while traveling

- **Stick to your routine:** Try to maintain your regular sleep, meal, and exercise routines as much as possible to minimize disruptions to your digestive system.
- **Plan your meals:** Research restaurants and grocery stores at your destination in advance to identify places that offer IBS-friendly food options. Pack some safe, non-perishable snacks for emergencies.

- **Stay hydrated:** Drinking enough water is crucial for digestive health. Carry a refillable water bottle with you and avoid consuming excessive amounts of caffeine or alcohol, which can exacerbate IBS symptoms.

- **Practice stress management:** Travel can be stressful, which may worsen IBS symptoms. Incorporate relaxation techniques, such as deep breathing, meditation, or gentle stretches, to help manage stress during your trip.

- **Pack a travel-sized IBS emergency kit:** Include items such as medication, a change of clothes, wet wipes, hand sanitizer, and a small pillow or cushion for added comfort during long journeys.

Preparing for travel with IBS

- **Consult your healthcare provider:** Discuss your travel plans and ask for any necessary medication adjustments or recommendations for managing your IBS symptoms while away from home.

- **Research your destination:** Familiarize yourself with the local cuisine and customs and the availability of restrooms and medical facilities.

- **Develop a meal plan:** Identify IBS-friendly dishes at your destination and plan your meals accordingly. Make a list of safe foods and ingredients to avoid.

- **Plan your itinerary with IBS in mind:** Schedule downtime for relaxation and self-care. Avoid overly ambitious itineraries that may exacerbate stress and IBS symptoms.

- **Consider travel insurance:** Invest in a comprehensive travel insurance policy that covers pre-existing conditions, including

IBS, to ensure you have access to medical care and support if needed during your trip.

Traveling with IBS may require some extra planning and preparation, but with the right strategies in place, you can enjoy your adventures without letting IBS hold you back. Prioritize your well-being and self-care, be prepared for unexpected situations, and embrace the opportunity to explore new places and create lasting memories.

IBS and Work

Managing your symptoms in a work environment can be demanding. However, by being proactive, open communication with your employer, and advocating for yourself, you can create a supportive and understanding workplace that helps you succeed.

Accommodations for people with IBS in the workplace

- **Flexible scheduling:** Arrange a flexible work schedule that allows for breaks or adjustments in your daily routine to accommodate your IBS symptoms.
- **Access to restrooms:** Request a workspace close to a restroom or ask permission to use restrooms on other floors or nearby buildings if necessary.
- **Remote work options:** In this post-pandemic world, remote work has become so much easier and more widely accepted. Discuss the possibility of working remotely or telecommuting full-time or on days when your IBS symptoms are particularly severe.
- **Modified work duties:** If specific job tasks exacerbate your IBS symptoms, explore the possibility of adjusting your responsibilities or swapping tasks with a coworker.

- **Break allowances:** Request additional breaks throughout the day to manage your symptoms, such as stretching, deep breathing, or using the restroom.

Talking to your employer about IBS

- **Choose the right time and place:** Schedule a private meeting with your supervisor to discuss your IBS and required accommodations.
- **Be prepared:** Research your workplace rights and have a list of possible accommodations ready to present during the conversation.
- **Be honest and concise:** Explain your IBS diagnosis, how it affects your daily life, and how it impacts your work.
- **Focus on solutions:** Emphasize your commitment to your job and present a plan to continue performing your duties with the requested accommodations.
- **Follow up in writing:** After your conversation, send a written summary of the discussion, including the agreed-upon accommodations, to both your supervisor and the human resources department.

Managing IBS symptoms at work

- **Prioritize self-care:** Practice stress management techniques, maintain a balanced diet, and exercise regularly to help control your IBS symptoms.
- **Plan your meals:** Bring IBS-friendly lunches and snacks to work to minimize the risk of triggering symptoms.
- **Establish a daily routine:** Develop a consistent daily routine incorporating breaks, meals, and relaxation techniques to help manage your symptoms.

- **Be prepared:** Keep a small emergency kit containing medication, extra clothing, and wet wipes at your workplace.
- **Seek support:** Connect with coworkers who may also be dealing with chronic health conditions and share experiences, strategies, and encouragement.

Disability benefits for people with IBS

- **Research your eligibility:** Investigate your eligibility for disability benefits or accommodations under laws such as the Americans with Disabilities Act (ADA) or the Family and Medical Leave Act (FMLA).
- **Consult with a healthcare professional:** Obtain a letter from your healthcare provider outlining your IBS diagnosis, its impact on your work, and any recommended accommodations.
- **Gather documentation:** Collect any relevant documentation, such as medical records, to support your request for disability benefits or accommodations.
- **Follow the application process:** Submit the necessary paperwork to apply for disability benefits or accommodations, adhering to deadlines and guidelines provided by your employer or the relevant government agency.
- **Seek legal advice if needed:** If you face resistance or discrimination in the workplace, consult with an attorney specializing in disability and employment law for guidance and support.

Navigating the workplace with IBS can be challenging, but by advocating for yourself and implementing the appropriate accommodations, you can create a supportive and understanding work environment. Stay proactive, prioritize self-care, and maintain open communication with your employer to ensure your ongoing success and well-being in the workplace.

Managing IBS in social settings

Living with IBS can sometimes make social situations more complicated. However, you can still enjoy a fulfilling social life with the right strategies. This section will cover managing your IBS symptoms while dining out, attending social events, and communicating with your loved ones about your condition.

Dining out with IBS

- **Plan ahead:** Before going to a restaurant, check their menu online to identify IBS-friendly options, or if needed, call ahead to discuss your dietary needs with the staff.
- **Make smart menu choices:** Opt for dishes with ingredients you know your body can tolerate. Avoid common IBS triggers like dairy, fatty or spicy foods, alcohol, and excessive caffeine.
- **Don't hesitate to ask:** Politely inquire about the ingredients in a dish. Don't be afraid to request modifications, such as swapping a side or leaving out a particular ingredient.
- **Eat slowly and mindfully:** Give your digestive system time to process your meal by eating slowly and chewing your food thoroughly.
- **Bring your snacks:** If you're unsure about the available options, bring your own IBS-friendly snacks to ensure you have something safe to eat.

Attending social events with IBS

- **Communicate your needs:** Let the event organizer or host know about your dietary restrictions in advance, so they can accommodate your needs if possible.
- **Be prepared:** Carry essential items such as medication, a change of clothes, and wet wipes in case you need them during the event.
- **Locate restrooms:** Discreetly find the nearest restroom upon arrival so you know where to go if needed.
- **Practice relaxation techniques:** Use deep breathing or visualization exercises to help manage stress and anxiety, which can exacerbate IBS symptoms.
- **Pace yourself:** Don't feel pressured to stay for the entire event. Listen to your body and leave when you feel it's necessary.

Embracing life with IBS doesn't mean you have to miss out on the experiences that make life enjoyable. By being proactive and prepared, you can continue to thrive in your work, travel, and social life. Communication, planning, and self-care are vital in managing your IBS symptoms and ensuring a fulfilling life. Stay optimistic, be patient, and surround yourself with supportive people who understand your journey. With the right mindset and strategies, you can confidently navigate life with IBS and create countless memories along the way.

Key Takeaways:

- Maintain regular sleep, meal, and exercise routines while traveling.
- Research and plan IBS-friendly meals in advance.
- Stay hydrated and practice stress management techniques.

- Pack a travel-sized IBS emergency kit.
- Consult a healthcare provider before traveling.
- Consider travel insurance that covers pre-existing conditions.
- Request workplace accommodations such as flexible scheduling and restroom access.
- Discuss remote work options with your employer.
- Be honest and concise when talking to your employer about IBS.
- Prioritize self-care and plan IBS-friendly meals at work.
- Research eligibility for disability benefits and accommodations.
- Plan ahead when dining out and make smart menu choices.
- Communicate dietary needs when attending social events.
- Practice relaxation techniques and pace yourself at events.

CHAPTER 15

Case Studies of Real-life Examples and Practical Solutions

"Experience is not what happens to you; it's what you do with what happens to you." – *Aldous Huxley*

Case Study 1:

Amanda is a 32-year-old teacher struggling with inconvenient and embarrassing symptoms including diarrhea, abdominal pain, and sudden need to use the bathroom during class. Her symptoms caused her to miss work and social events, leaving her frustrated and isolated. Despite eliminating dairy and gluten from her diet, Amanda's symptoms persisted. She was open to trying other options, like medication and stress management techniques.

After running some tests, I diagnosed Amanda with IBS-D based on her symptoms.

Strategies for managing symptoms:

- Suggested Amanda try a low FODMAP diet
- Probiotics (Align) daily

Follow-up after 4 weeks:

She felt a bit better when she returned, but her symptoms hadn't completely disappeared. She still had a sudden urge to use the bathroom after eating. I offered her a few options, including antidepressants and Xifaxan, and she decided to try antidepressants.

- Prescribed her 25 mg of desipramine to be taken at bedtime
- Recommended that she see a psychologist or try online therapy for cognitive behavioral therapy.

Follow-up after 2 months:

Amanda felt much better on desipramine but decided not to pursue CBT because she found it too expensive. Since she tolerated the desipramine well, I advised her to continue taking it long-term. Meanwhile, I suggested she slowly reintroduce some FODMAP foods and keep a food diary to track her reactions and identify triggers.

Follow-up after 6 months:

At her six-month follow-up, Amanda was still doing well. She had reintroduced most foods except dairy, onions, and garlic. She was thrilled with her progress.

Case Study 2:

Carmen is a 45-year-old woman who has been experiencing symptoms including diarrhea, bloating, and abdominal pain for two years. She's noticed her symptoms worsen during stressful times, which are frequent due to her demanding job as an executive. After ordering some tests, I found nothing abnormal, only a few polyps during her colonoscopy.

Strategies for managing symptoms:

- Recommended that Carmen try a lactose-free diet
- Discussed with her about managing stress with techniques like yoga, deep breathing, meditation, and exercise.

- Imodium is to be taken as needed for diarrhea, especially when traveling.

<u>Follow-up after 2 months:</u>

When Carmen returned for a follow-up after two months, she was doing much better on the lactose-free diet. She had switched to oat milk and avoided cheese and ice cream as much as possible. She also started attending spinning classes three times a week, which helped her manage stress more effectively. Overall, she was feeling much better.

Case Study 3:

Nicole is a 55-year-old woman who's been dealing with constipation, abdominal cramping and bloating for several years. She was hesitant to take medication due to concerns about side effects. Nicole had some tests done, like blood count and thyroid function, which came back normal. Her colonoscopy was also normal.

<u>Strategies for managing symptoms:</u>

I talked to Nicole about IBS, its natural history, various dietary options, medications, etc. Since her symptoms were mild, I didn't think she needed prescription medications.

- MiraLAX three times a week at bedtime,
- Gas-X is to be taken as needed for bloating.
- Recommended that she cut back on dairy products, raw vegetables, and salads.
- Try some relaxation techniques like deep breathing or meditation.

Follow-up after 3 months:

When Nicole returned for a follow-up after three months, her bloating had improved, but she still had constipation. She was trying meditation but not sticking to it consistently. I suggested she increase Mira-LAX to daily use and try speed walking to see if it would help.

Follow-up after 2 months:

Two months later, Nicole's constipation had improved with MiraLAX, and she had started speed walking three miles a day, about three times a week, on a trail near her home. Overall, she was pleased with her progress.

Case Study 4:

Albert is a 45-year-old construction worker struggling with IBS-C symptoms like constipation, bloating, and abdominal pain for more than 6 months. These issues seem to improve after he has a bowel movement, but they've made him miss work and worry about his ability to keep doing his physically demanding job. He's tried changing his diet and increasing fiber, but his symptoms haven't improved. Albert wants to explore other treatment options, including medications. Albert's tests, including blood work and a colonoscopy, were normal.

Strategies for managing symptoms:

- Follow a lactose-free diet
- Start taking Senokot, 1 to 2 tablets every night at bedtime.

Follow-up after 1 month:

After a month, Albert was still experiencing significant abdominal discomfort and bloating. His constipation had improved, but he still felt he wasn't fully emptying his bowels.

At this point-

- Prescribed Linzess 145 mcg to be taken in the evening after he gets home. He called back after a week, saying Linzess was causing uncontrollable diarrhea, so I gave him samples of Linzess 72 mcg to try.

Follow-up after 6 weeks:

At his 6-week follow-up, Albert was doing much better, with significant improvement in abdominal discomfort, bloating, and constipation. He no longer had diarrhea when taking Linzess.

Case Study 5:

Maria is a 35-year-old woman who is 24 weeks pregnant with her first child. She's had IBS-D and worries about how her symptoms might affect her pregnancy. Since becoming pregnant, her heartburn has gotten worse. Maria has been experiencing diarrhea 2-3 times daily, usually right after a meal. She's tried to manage her symptoms by avoiding trigger foods like spicy and fried foods, which has helped her heartburn but not her other symptoms. She's also interested in exploring other safe treatment options during pregnancy. When I saw Maria, she brought in blood work from her obstetrician, which included blood count, thyroid function, and stool tests which were all normal.

Strategies for managing symptoms:

I talked to Maria about IBS, its natural history, and treatment options. I also reassured her that IBS is a benign condition and shouldn't affect her baby. I suggested:

- A low FODMAP diet
- Avoid raw vegetables and salads.

- Recommended yoga or other relaxation techniques to help manage stress, which can worsen IBS symptoms.

Follow-up after 4 weeks:

When I saw her for a follow-up, she was doing much better, with less abdominal pain and diarrhea. I told her to slowly reintroduce FOD-MAP foods and see how she tolerates them to identify triggers. Maria did well throughout her pregnancy and delivered a healthy baby. She continues to follow the diet and lifestyle changes for IBS with good results.

Case Study 6:

Martha is a 70-year-old woman who's been struggling with IBS for quite some time. Lately, she's been struggling with constipation, experiencing lower belly cramps that go away after she she has a bowel movement. She only manages to go 3-4 times a week, and it's always a strain. To make matters worse, she's dealing with bloating and lots of gas. I reviewed all her test results and recent colonoscopy report, and everything was normal.

Strategies for managing symptoms:

- Eat more soluble fiber, drink more water
- Take a tablespoon of Metamucil at bedtime
- Cut down on dairy
- Try an over-the-counter supplement with probiotics, prebiotics, and digestive enzymes (IBplus).
- Deep breathing exercises and adding physical activity to her daily routine.

Follow-up after 2 months:

Her constipation and bloating had greatly improved, and she was thrilled with the results.

Case Study 7:

Maya is a 27-year-old woman who has been dealing with IBS symptoms for the past two years. She often experiences bloating, belly pain, and diarrhea after eating certain foods. She said, "I feel like I have a big rock in my belly." Despite trying to identify her triggers, she has had no success. She feels frustrated with her symptoms, making her feel like she can no longer enjoy eating.

Maya is otherwise healthy and has no other medical issues. She works as a software consultant and leads a low-stress lifestyle. She attends hot yoga classes four times a week. She has no family history of inflammatory bowel disease or celiac disease.

Strategies for managing symptoms:

I spoke with Maya about IBS-D, dietary triggers, and medications. Since Maya did not want to rely on long-term medications for her IBS, I suggested a low-FODMAP diet and provided instructions on how to follow it. I also recommended that she download the Monash FODMAP diet app to help her track food triggers. Additionally, I prescribed a 14-day course of Xifaxan 550 mg three times a day to help her manage her symptoms.

Follow-up after 3 months:

When I saw Maya after three months, she was doing much better. Maya had identified and eliminated some dietary triggers, improving her overall health. I reminded her that IBS is a lifelong condition that requires ongoing management. I advised her to continue following the diet and gave her the option of using antibiotics as needed in the future.

Case Study 8:

Abdul, a 46-year-old man, has been dealing with extreme diarrhea, belly pain, and bloating for over a year. He's recently been diagnosed with IBS by his primary care provider. Despite trying elimination diets and various over-the-counter medications, Abdul's symptoms persist, and he's worried about their impact on his work and social life. Abdul is otherwise healthy, with no family history of celiac disease, Crohn's, or ulcerative colitis. He's never had any issues with his gallbladder. I reviewed the blood tests, and stool panel results that his primary care provider ordered, and everything looked normal. A colonoscopy revealed one polyp but no signs of colitis.

Strategies for managing symptoms:

Considering his significant symptoms and their effect on his life, I recommended we treat Abdul more aggressively.

- A low FODMAP diet
- Started him on Eluxadoline (Viberzi).
- Recommended gut-directed hypnotherapy.

Follow-up after 3 months:

When I saw Abdul again after three months, his symptoms were much more manageable. He had just finished a 12-week gut-directed hypnotherapy. His diarrhea had significantly reduced, and his belly pain and bloating had entirely resolved. I advised him to slowly reintroduce FODMAP-containing foods while keeping a food diary to identify triggers. I recommended that he continue Viberzi. Abdul continues to do well.

Case Study 9:

Laura is a 40-year-old woman with constant bloating and occasional belly pain, sometimes developing severe cramps if she's not careful with certain foods. She also has on-and-off diarrhea when eating specific foods, which she tries to avoid. Apart from gastric bypass surgery in the past, she's in good health.

Laura was diagnosed with IBS by her primary care provider. Her primary care provider suggested she try cutting out common food triggers like lactose and fructose from her diet. This helped with her diarrhea, but her bloating remained an issue. She still had episodes of abdominal pain when she was not careful with her diet.

Strategies for managing symptoms:

Given her previous history of surgery, I suspected that Laura might have small intestinal bacterial overgrowth (SIBO). At this point, we could either do a breath test or try antibiotic therapy. We chose to proceed with antibiotics.

- Prescribed doxycycline (100 mg twice a day for 10 days)
- Levsin, a medication that she can take under her tongue only when needed for abdominal pain.
- Stress reduction techniques like deep breathing exercises and mindfulness meditation.

Follow-up after 3 months:

She downloaded an app for mindfulness meditation which she found useful. Her bloating had significantly improved, and her occasional belly pain had become much less frequent. She had to take Levsin only few times.

Case Study 10:

Bill is a 70-year-old retiree who used to work as a bank manager. He's lived with IBS since his 30s, but his symptoms were mild until recently. Lately, he's been experiencing lower belly cramps after meals and a frequent urge to use the bathroom. He's been struggling with periods of both diarrhea and constipation. Bill tried a lactose-free diet, but it didn't help much.

Sadly, Bill lost his wife about a year ago and has been living alone since then. He feels lonely and anxious about the future, which contributed to his symptoms. I checked Bill's blood work with his primary care physician and found them to be normal. I also reviewed his colonoscopy report from a year ago, showing that he had a few polyps removed.

Strategies for managing symptoms:

We chatted about IBS-M, its natural history, common triggers, and treatment options like hypnotherapy, CBT, and medications. Bill wasn't interested in psychotherapy or seeing a psychiatrist but agreed to meet with a counselor.

- Prescribed an antidepressant, Paroxetine 20 mg, to take daily at bedtime.

- Avoid dairy, raw vegetables, and salads.

- Incorporate physical activity into his daily routine.

Follow-up after 2 months:

Bill started going to the YMCA, doing strength training exercises, and using the elliptical machine 2-3 times a week. He felt much better overall, tolerating Paroxetine without any side effects. Talking to the counselor had made a positive impact on his well-being.

It is important to keep in mind that what may have worked for one patient with IBS may not necessarily work for another. IBS is a complicated condition with various symptoms that can appear in different combinations and intensities in different individuals. Additionally, each person may have a specific symptom that they want to target or a specific type of treatment that they prefer. To find the most effective treatment plan, people with IBS should work together with their healthcare provider to create a personalized approach that caters to their individual needs and circumstances.

CHAPTER 16

Future Directions in
IBS Research and Treatment

*"Research is to see what everybody else has seen, and to think what
nobody else has thought." - Albert Szent-Györgyi*

The world of IBS research is growing fast. Scientists are constantly
making new discoveries, trying to figure out IBS's mysteries, and
developing better treatments. Let's explore some of these exciting discoveries and see what the future will bring to make the management
of IBS better.

New clues to IBS causes

Researchers are studying many possible reasons for IBS, like genes,
changes in gut bacteria, immune system problems, and how the gut
and brain communicate. As we learn more, our understanding of IBS
keeps getting better.

Sunshine vitamin and feel-good brain chemicals

Vitamin D, the sunshine vitamin, and mood-boosting brain chemicals
like serotonin and brain-derived neurotrophic factor (BDNF) might
help people with IBS, especially those dealing with diarrhea and stress.
Keeping an eye on these essential elements could lead to better IBS
management and personalized treatments.

Bile acids and gut bacteria: a crucial conversation

Research shows that the connection between bile acids and gut bacteria play a significant role in IBS. This connection leads to changes in gut bacteria, bile acid pathways, and bacterial by-products. Studying how different bile acid profiles affect the gut could help us understand their role in IBS and lead to targeted treatments.

Tryptophan: connecting the gut and brain

An exciting area of research is looking at the gut-brain axis, which shows how our gut bacteria affect our brain and behavior. Tryptophan, an essential amino acid, seems to be a crucial link in this connection, opening up fascinating possibilities for understanding our health.

Bacterial proteases: small enzymes, with a big impact

Proteases are enzymes that break down proteins and play an essential role in digestion and inflammation. Keeping a balance between proteases and their targets is vital for gut health. Learning more about these enzymes could lead to new treatments for common gut issues.

Epigenetics and IBS

Epigenetics is the study of changes in how genes work that aren't caused by changes in the DNA itself. Factors like diet, stress, and toxins can influence these changes. Researchers now find that epigenetics may also play a role in IBS, adding to our understanding of this complex condition.

New ways to diagnose IBS

New tools like breath tests, biomarkers, and advanced imaging techniques are being developed to make it easier to diagnose IBS.

Biomarkers: predicting IBS

Biomarkers are substances in the body that can be measured to show the presence of a specific condition. Scientists are studying different biomarkers for IBS, like blood and stool tests that can find inflammation or changes in gut bacteria. We are still learning about these biomarkers, but the progress is promising. As we learn more, personalized care for IBS patients could become the norm, leading to better treatments and improved quality of life.

Advanced imaging techniques: a clearer picture of the gut

Regular imaging techniques like X-rays or ultrasounds might not help diagnose IBS, but newer methods like MRI can give detailed images of the gut and show how food moves through the digestive system. This information could help doctors tell IBS apart from other gut issues.

Neuroimaging: seeing the gut-brain connection

As we learn more about how the gut and brain communicate in IBS, neuroimaging techniques like functional MRI (fMRI) are being studied for their potential to diagnose IBS. These methods can show brain activity in response to gut signals helping doctors understand the gut-brain connection and spot disruptions that might be causing IBS symptoms.

Machine learning and artificial intelligence: High-tech IBS diagnosis

By combining data from symptoms, blood tests, and imaging studies, machine learning and artificial intelligence (AI) could find patterns that set IBS apart from other conditions with similar symptoms. AI can even help endoscopy cameras in the colon detect specific signs of IBS. While this technology is still developing, it could play a significant role in diagnosing IBS in the future.

Personalized medicine

The gut microbiome is a hot topic in IBS research. Studies are examining how imbalances in gut bacteria might cause IBS symptoms. Potential treatments like probiotics, prebiotics, and fecal microbiota transplantation (FMT) are being explored.

The gut-brain connection

By now, you have come across the gut-brain connection so many times in this book which shows how important it is in IBS. Scientists are now studying how the microbiome affects this connection and its role in IBS symptoms. This research might lead to new therapies customized to our specific gut and brain profiles, offering a more comprehensive approach to managing IBS.

Personalized medicine tailored to your gut bacteria

Researchers use high-tech methods to study the trillions of bacteria living in our guts as we learn more about the gut microbiome's role in IBS. This could lead to personalized treatments based on your unique gut bacteria, offering more targeted and effective IBS therapies. Seed Health (https://seed.com/) and Viome (https://www.viome.com/) are examples of companies that analyze your gut microbiome using advanced DNA sequencing technology. They provide personalized recommendations to improve your gut health.

The genetic connection

Researchers have suspected that genetics play a role in IBS, and recent studies support this idea. Scientists can better understand complex genetic factors by identifying specific genes linked to IBS. This knowledge could lead to targeted therapies based on an individual's unique genetic makeup, and gene-editing technologies like CRISPR/Cas9 could someday help treat or prevent IBS.

As we learn more about the genetic and epigenetic factors involved in IBS, personalized medicine becomes a reality. Analyzing an individual's genetic profile could help doctors find the most effective therapies for that person, revolutionizing IBS treatment with customized solutions that provide better results and fewer side effects.

Dietary approaches for IBS

Emerging dietary interventions for IBS include personalized nutrition plans based on an individual's unique gut microbiome profile and the use of nutraceuticals, which are natural compounds with potential health benefits for IBS sufferers.

Personalized nutrition

Personalized nutrition is gaining attention as a possible IBS management strategy. Healthcare professionals can create tailored meal plans by analyzing a person's genetic makeup, gut bacteria, and individual food sensitivities. Some small studies show that AI can design diets based on individual gut microbiome features, improving IBS-related symptoms.

Psychobiotics

Psychobiotics are a new class of probiotics that can potentially influence brain function and mood through the gut-brain axis. Certain strains of beneficial bacteria, such as Bifidobacterium and Lactobacillus, show promise in improving IBS symptoms and overall well-being. Consuming psychobiotic-rich foods like yogurt and kefir or taking probiotic supplements might help some people with IBS.

Polyphenols

These are natural compounds found in plant-based foods with anti-oxidant and anti-inflammatory properties. Recent research suggests that polyphenols may positively impact gut health and IBS symptoms. Incorporating polyphenol-rich foods like berries, dark chocolate, and green tea into your diet may help improve gut function and reduce IBS symptoms.

Psychological therapies for IBS relief

Mindfulness-oriented recovery enhancement (MORE)

MORE is a newer integrative psychological therapy that combines mindfulness, cognitive-behavioral therapy, and positive psychology principles. MORE has been initially developed for treating chronic pain and opioid misuse, improving pain symptoms, emotional regulation, and well-being. It might hold promise for IBS patients, as the therapy targets pain and emotional regulation, critical factors in IBS.

Biofeedback

With biofeedback, patients can learn to master bodily processes like heart rate, muscle tension, and bowel function. Patients learn to interpret their body's signals and adjust to minimize IBS symptoms using sensors and visual or auditory feedback. Newer biofeedback devices and applications are making this therapy more accessible and user-friendly.

Immune-based therapies: exciting developments

Scientists are unlocking the connection between the immune system and IBS, leading to new treatments targeting the condition's root cause.

Tackling inflammation

Some IBS patients have low-grade gut inflammation. Researchers are exploring treatments, like medications and natural compounds, to reduce inflammation and ease IBS symptoms.

Mast cell stabilizers

Mast cells release chemicals causing inflammation and pain in IBS. By stabilizing these cells, new therapies aim to reduce symptoms. One promising medication is ketotifen, a medication that is primarily used to treat allergies such as hay fever and eye allergies.

Probiotics

Beneficial bacteria can help regulate the immune system and lower inflammation. Specific probiotics, like Bifidobacterium infantis and Lactobacillus plantarum, may improve IBS symptoms. Expect more targeted probiotic treatments as research continues.

Some of these therapies are still experimental, but they offer a brighter future for IBS management and patients' quality of life.

Neurostimulation therapies: the cutting-edge frontier

Neurostimulation therapies use electrical or magnetic impulses to stimulate nerves or brain areas, improving IBS symptoms by regulating the gut-brain axis.

Vagus nerve stimulation (VNS)

The vagus nerve connects the brain and digestive system. VNS uses electrical stimulation to target this nerve, alleviating IBS symptoms. Currently used for epilepsy and depression, it could also help manage IBS.

Transcranial magnetic stimulation (TMS)

A non-invasive therapy using magnetic fields to stimulate specific brain areas. Targeting regions involved in pain processing and the gut-brain axis may reduce IBS pain and improve symptoms. Though primarily used for depression, TMS is being studied as a potential IBS treatment.

These emerging neurostimulation therapies provide a glimpse into the future of IBS treatment, where non-invasive, targeted solutions could transform the lives of those affected. While more research is needed, their potential to revolutionize IBS management brings hope to patients seeking relief.

Digital technology to the rescue: a glimpse into the future of IBS management

Digital technology is making life easier for those affected by IBS. Let's dive into the world of smart apps, wearable technology, and virtual reality, transforming IBS management and brightening the future!

Smartphone apps

With an app for almost everything, IBS management has become simpler. Track your symptoms, identify triggers, and find personalized meal plans, low-FODMAP recipes, and stress-reducing exercises – all in one place!

Wearable technology

Smartwatches and fitness trackers now monitor health aspects like sleep, stress, and physical activity. By monitoring these factors, you can identify patterns and make lifestyle changes to improve your IBS.

Telemedicine

Virtual consultations with healthcare professionals mean easier access to specialists like gastroenterologists and dietitians without long waits or travel. This is especially helpful for those in remote areas or with limited mobility.

Digital cognitive behavioral therapy (CBT)

Digital CBT programs, available through apps and websites, bring psychological support to your fingertips, making it more accessible and convenient for IBS patients.

Virtual Reality (VR): a new frontier for IBS relief

Imagine stepping into a vivid, three-dimensional world that takes you away from your IBS symptoms. VR creates immersive environments that feel incredibly real, responding to your head movements to adjust visuals.

Since the brain-gut connection influences IBS, treatments targeting the central nervous system can help ease symptoms. Traditional therapies like CBT and hypnotherapy are helpful, but finding a suitable therapist and managing costs and accessibility can be challenging.

A 2022 study explored a unique VR program for IBS, featuring immersive experiences about the brain-gut axis, IBS-specific CBT, gut-directed meditation, and a module addressing social isolation and stigma. While still in its early stages, this promising technology could revolutionize IBS treatment.

The buzzing pill: a new approach to treatment

In the world of innovative treatments, abdominal physical stimulation is gaining attention. The vibrating capsule, a non-drug solution, is a small, programmable pill you swallow. It buzzes inside your body to trigger bowel movements. It has proven effective for those with constipation. Although there are no studies yet showing its effectiveness in IBS patients, it might be a potential treatment for people with IBS-C.

In summary, the future of IBS research and treatment is filled with exciting possibilities. As we learn more about this complex condition, our ability to diagnose, manage, and improve the lives of those living with IBS will only improve. The future of IBS management is brighter than ever, thanks to rapid technological advancements. With smart apps, wearable devices, telemedicine, and personalized treatments becoming more accessible and convenient, we can look forward to even more groundbreaking innovations to improve the lives of IBS sufferers worldwide.

CHAPTER 17

Conclusion

"Embracing the journey of IBS means discovering the harmony between mind, body, and gut – a symphony of hope, resilience, and healing."

Let's wrap up our IBS journey by reviewing key points and exploring how a holistic integrated approach can make living with IBS easier. With the right mindset, body awareness, and support, managing IBS can be less of a challenge.

Recap of key takeaways from the book

1. IBS is a common but complex gut problem affecting millions. It causes abdominal pain, bloating, and changes in bowel movements like diarrhea or constipation.

2. IBS causes are unclear, but factors include gut-brain interaction, genetics, gut sensitivity, an imbalance in gut bacteria, and stress.

3. Proper diagnosis is crucial, so work with healthcare professionals to create a personal treatment plan.

4. Diet, lifestyle, and stress management are vital in managing IBS, and everyone's journey is different.

5. Currently, therapies such as CBT and hypnotherapy are not being used enough, even though they have the potential to assist many patients.

6. In cases where natural therapies like dietary changes, lifestyle adjustments, and stress reduction techniques are not successful in alleviating symptoms, there are various medications available for individuals with IBS.

7. New research and treatments are giving hope to people with IBS. Knowing how the brain and gut work together, the role of gut bacteria, and exploring new ways to treat IBS can make life better for those dealing with this condition.

Final thoughts on living with IBS

Living with IBS can be challenging, but being proactive and embracing a whole-body approach can help manage symptoms and leads to a happier life. Remember, self-care, stress management, and emotional support are essential for your well-being. Be patient and compassionate with yourself as you try new strategies or treatments.

As someone living with IBS or supporting a loved one, it is essential to raise awareness about the condition by sharing your story and educating others. Participating in local events and engaging with online communities can contribute to the collective effort to improve the understanding and management of IBS.

Patient-centered integrated care is the future of IBS care

The future of IBS treatment lies in patient-centered care, which takes into account each individual's unique experience and needs. This approach can lead to personalized treatment plans, better doctor-patient communication, a holistic approach to care for empowered patients, and collaborative care among healthcare professionals.

The shift towards patient-centered care is a promising and exciting change in IBS treatment. As research advances, this approach will become more critical, offering hope and better outcomes for those living with IBS.

Resources for further reading and support

1. American College of Gastroenterology: A professional organization for gastroenterologists that offers resources and information on gastrointestinal disorders, including IBS. IBS-specific information: https://gi.org/topics/irritable-bowel-syndrome/

2. Rome Foundation: An organization dedicated to improving the lives of people with functional gastrointestinal disorders like IBS through research and education. IBS-specific information: https://theromefoundation.org/rome-iv/functional-gastrointestinal-disorders/irritable-bowel-syndrome/

3. International Foundation for Gastrointestinal Disorders (IFFGD): https://www.iffgd.org/

4. About IBS: A resource provided by the IFFGD that offers comprehensive information on IBS, including diagnosis, treatment, and management. https://aboutibs.org/

5. Academy of Nutrition and Dietetics: https://www.eatright.org/

6. National Institute of Diabetes and Digestive and Kidney Diseases (NIDDK): https://www.niddk.nih.gov/

I hope that this book has equipped you with valuable knowledge and tools to understand and manage your IBS. Remember that you're not alone. Stay informed, be proactive, and embrace a holistic approach to living with IBS. Together, we can make a difference in the lives of those affected. Stay optimistic as researchers work hard to find better ways to manage IBS and improve patients' quality of life. The future of living with IBS is looking brighter and more manageable than ever before!

CHAPTER 18

28-day Low-FODMAP Diet Plan with Full Recipes

Day 1

Day 1- Breakfast: Low-FODMAP Blueberry Pancakes

Description: Start your day with delicious blueberry pancakes that are low in FODMAPs and easy to make.

Preparation and Cooking Time: 20 minutes

Number of Servings: 2

Ingredients:

- 1 cup gluten-free flour
- 1 tbsp granulated sugar
- 2 tsp baking powder
- 1/4 tsp salt
- 3 tbsp lactose-free milk
- 1 large egg
- 1 tbsp vegetable oil
- 1/2 cup fresh blueberries
- Maple syrup or LOW FODMAP jam (optional)

Directions:

- Whisk together flour, sugar, baking powder, and salt in a large bowl.
- In a separate bowl, whisk together milk, egg, and vegetable oil.

- Pour the wet ingredients into the dry ingredients and stir until combined.
- Gently fold in the blueberries.
- Preheat a non-stick skillet over medium heat.
- Scoop 1/4 cup of batter onto the skillet and cook for 2-3 minutes until bubbles form on the surface.
- Flip the pancake and cook for an additional 1-2 minutes.
- Repeat with the remaining batter.
- Serve warm with maple syrup or a low-FODMAP jam.

Substitution ideas: You can use rice flour, or potato starch as your gluten-free flour. You can replace lactose-free milk with plant-based milk such as almond or soy milk (made from isolated soy proteins). You may opt for strawberry or blueberry as your low-FODMAP jam.

In choosing a Low-FODMAP jam, check the ingredient's nutrition label list for fructose syrup or honey since these ingredients have high FODMAP content.

Nutrition Information (per serving excluding the maple syrup or jam): Calories:366, Protein: 10.2g, Fat: 11g, Carbohydrates: 59g, Fiber: 7g, Sugar: 10.9g

Day 1-Lunch: Grilled Chicken Salad with Lemon-Tahini Dressing

Description: A fresh, flavorful salad with grilled chicken and a tangy low-FODMAP lemon-tahini dressing.

Preparation and Cooking Time: 30 minutes

Number of Servings: 2

Ingredients:

- ½ lb or 2 boneless, skinless chicken breasts
- Salt and pepper, to taste
- 4 cups mixed salad greens
- 1/2 cup cherry tomatoes, halved
- 1/4 cup cucumber, sliced
- 1/4 cup red bell pepper, sliced
- 2 tbsp walnuts, chopped

For the Lemon-Tahini Dressing:

- 1/4 cup tahini
- 2/3 pc lemon, juiced
- 2 tbsp garlic-infused olive oil
- 2 tbsp water
- Salt, to taste

Directions:

- Preheat a grill or grill pan over medium heat.
- Season chicken breasts with salt and pepper, then grill for 6-7 minutes per side, or until cooked through. Set aside to cool.
- Combine salad greens, cherry tomatoes, cucumber, and red bell pepper in a large salad bowl.
- Slice the cooled chicken and add to the salad.
- In a small bowl, whisk together tahini, lemon juice, garlic-infused olive oil, water, and salt to make the dressing.
- Drizzle the dressing over the salad and toss to combine.
- Top with chopped walnuts and serve.

Nutrition Information (per serving):   Calories: 512, Protein: 37.2g, Fat: 34.1g, Carbohydrates: 20.8g, Fiber: 4g, Sugar: 2.6g

Day 1-Dinner: Low-FODMAP Shrimp Stir-Fry

Description: An easy and flavorful shrimp stir-fry with colorful veggies that's perfect for a low-FODMAP diet.

Preparation and Cooking Time: 25 minutes

Number of Servings: 2

Ingredients:

- 8 oz shrimp, peeled and deveined
- 1 tbsp garlic-infused olive oil
- 1/2 cup red bell pepper, sliced
- 1/2 cup zucchini, sliced
- 1/2 cup carrots, julienned
- 2 tbsp soy sauce (gluten-free)
- 1 tbsp fresh ginger, grated
- 2 green onions (green tops only), sliced
- Salt and pepper, to taste
- 2 cups cooked white rice

Directions:

- Heat garlic-infused olive oil in a large skillet over medium heat.
- Add shrimp to the skillet and cook for 2-3 minutes per side until pink and cooked through. Transfer shrimp to a plate and set aside.
- In the same skillet, add red bell pepper, zucchini, and carrots. Cook for 5-7 minutes, stirring occasionally, until the vegetables are tender.
- In a small bowl, combine soy sauce and grated ginger.
- Add the cooked shrimp back to the skillet with the vegetables.
- Pour the soy sauce mixture over the shrimp and vegetables and stir to combine.
- Cook for an additional 1-2 minutes, then remove from heat.
- Season with salt and pepper, then top with green onion slices.
- Serve over cooked white rice.

Nutrition Information (per serving): Calories: 443, Protein: 29g, Fat: 8.7g, Carbohydrates: 62.3g, Fiber: 2.7g, Sugar: 3.8g

Day 2

Day 2 - Breakfast: Low-FODMAP Banana Pancakes

Description: Fluffy, gluten-free pancakes made with ripe bananas and topped with maple syrup.

Preparation and Cooking Time: 20 minutes

Number of Servings: 2 Serving Size: 2 pancakes

Ingredients:

- 1 "just ripe" banana, mashed
- 2 large eggs
- 1/2 cup gluten-free flour
- 1/2 tsp baking powder
- Pinch of salt
- 1/4 tsp cinnamon
- 1 tsp vanilla extract
- 2 tbsp lactose-free milk
- Cooking spray or oil for greasing
- 2 tbsp maple syrup, for serving

Directions:

- In a mixing bowl, combine the mashed banana, eggs, gluten-free flour, baking powder, salt, cinnamon, vanilla extract, and lactose-free milk. Mix until smooth. 2. Preheat a non-stick skillet or griddle over medium heat and lightly grease with cooking spray or oil.

- Pour 1/4 cup of the batter onto the skillet for each pancake. Cook until bubbles appear on the surface and the edges begin to set about 2-3 minutes. Flip the pancake and cook for another 1-2 minutes until golden brown.
- Serve the pancakes with maple syrup.

Substitution ideas: You can use rice flour, or potato starch as your gluten-free flour. You can replace lactose-free milk with plant-based milk such as almond or soy milk (made from isolated soy proteins).

Nutrition Information (per serving): Calories:238, Protein: 7.3g, Fat: 3.9g, Carbohydrates: 44.3g, Fiber: 4.7g, Sugar: 14.4g

Day 2 - Lunch: Low-FODMAP Egg Salad Lettuce Wraps

Description: A light and refreshing lunch featuring a creamy egg salad served in crisp lettuce wraps.

Preparation and Cooking Time: 20 minutes

Number of Servings: 2

Ingredients:

- 4 hard-boiled eggs, peeled and chopped
- 1/4 cup plain mayonnaise
- 1 tbsp Dijon mustard
- 1 tbsp chives, chopped
- Salt and pepper, to taste
- 4 large lettuce leaves, (iceberg or butter lettuce)

Directions:

- In a medium bowl, combine chopped hard-boiled eggs, mayonnaise, Dijon mustard, and chives.
- Season with salt and pepper, and mix well.
- Divide the egg salad mixture evenly among the 4 lettuce leaves.
- Fold the lettuce leaves around the egg salad to create wraps and serve.

Note: In choosing mayonnaise, check the ingredient's nutrition label list. Watch out for onion or garlic since these ingredients have high FODMAP content.

Nutrition Information (per serving): Calories: 336, Protein: 11.6g, Fat: 31.1g, Carbohydrates: 2.1g, Fiber: 0.5g, Sugar: 1.1g

Day 2 - Dinner: Low-FODMAP Lemon-Herb Baked Salmon

Description: Flavorful and tender baked salmon with a zesty lemon-herb topping that's perfect for a low-FODMAP diet.

Preparation and Cooking Time: 30 minutes

Number of Servings: 2

Ingredients:

- 2 (6 oz each) salmon fillets
- Salt and pepper, to taste
- 2 tbsp garlic-infused olive oil
- 1/3 pc lemon, juiced
- 1 tbsp fresh parsley, chopped
- 1 tsp fresh dill, chopped
- 1 tsp lemon zest
- 2 cups quinoa, cooked

Directions:

- Preheat oven to 400°F (200°C) and line a baking sheet with parchment paper.
- Place salmon fillets on the prepared baking sheet and season with salt and pepper.
- In a small bowl, combine garlic-infused olive oil, lemon juice, parsley, dill, and lemon zest.
- Spoon the herb mixture evenly over the salmon fillets.
- Bake for 12-15 minutes or until the salmon flakes easily with a fork.
- Serve the salmon over cooked quinoa.

Nutrition Information (per serving): Calories: 635, Protein: 51.7g, Fat: 30.8g, Carbohydrates: 39.8g, Fiber: 5.2g, Sugar: 0.2g

Day 3

Day 3-Breakfast: Low-FODMAP Spinach and Feta Frittata

Description: A delicious and easy-to-make frittata packed with spinach, feta cheese, and fresh herbs.

Preparation and Cooking Time: 40 minutes

Number of Servings: 4 Serving Size: 1/4 of the frittata

Ingredients:

- 8 large eggs
- 1/4 cup lactose-free milk
- Salt and pepper, to taste
- 1 tbsp olive oil

- 1/2 cup green onions (green tops only), chopped
- 2 cups packed baby spinach
- 1/2 cup feta cheese, crumbled
- 1/4 cup fresh basil, chopped

Directions:

- Preheat the oven to 350°F (180°C).
- In a bowl, whisk together the eggs, lactose-free milk, salt, and pepper.
- Heat the olive oil in a 10-inch ovenproof skillet over medium heat. Add the scallions and cook for 1-2 minutes until softened.
- Add the spinach and cook until wilted, about 2-3 minutes.
- Pour the egg mixture into the skillet and cook for 2-3 minutes until the edges start to set. Sprinkle the feta cheese and basil on top.
- Transfer the skillet to the oven and bake for 15-20 minutes until the frittata is cooked through and the top is golden.

Substitution ideas: You can replace lactose-free milk with plant-based milk such as almond or soy milk (made from isolated soy proteins).

Nutrition Information (per serving):   Calories: 255, Protein: 17g, Fat: 17.8g, Carbohydrates: 8.3g, Fiber: 2.9g, Sugar: 2.6g

Day 3 - Lunch: Low-FODMAP Chicken, Quinoa, and Veggie Bowl

Description: A nourishing and flavorful bowl filled with grilled chicken, quinoa, and colorful veggies, perfect for a low-FODMAP lunch.

Preparation and Cooking Time: 30 minutes

Number of Servings: 2

Ingredients:

- ½ lb or 2 boneless, skinless chicken breasts
- Salt and pepper, to taste
- 1 tbsp garlic-infused olive oil
- 2 cups quinoa, cooked
- 1 cup cherry tomatoes, halved
- 1/2 cup cucumber, diced
- 1/4 cup green onions (green tops only), sliced
- 1/4 cup fresh cilantro, chopped
- 1 1/3 pc lemon, juiced
- 1/4 cup feta cheese, crumbled

Directions:

- Preheat the grill or grill pan to medium-high heat.
- Season chicken breasts with salt and pepper.
- Grill chicken breasts for 5-7 minutes per side or until cooked through. Let rest for a few minutes, then slice into strips.
- In a large bowl, combine cooked quinoa, cherry tomatoes, cucumber, scallions, cilantro, and lemon juice. Mix well.
- Divide quinoa mixture between two bowls, then top with grilled chicken strips.
- Sprinkle with feta cheese and serve.

Nutrition Information (per serving): Calories: 484, Protein: 38.1g, Fat: 17g, Carbohydrates: 45.9g, Fiber: 6.7g, Sugar: 4.5g

Day 3 - Dinner: Low-FODMAP Shrimp Stir-Fry with Rice Noodles

Description: A quick and easy shrimp stir-fry with colorful veggies and rice noodles for a satisfying low-FODMAP dinner.

Preparation and Cooking Time: 30 minutes

Number of Servings: 2

Ingredients:

- 4 oz rice noodles
- 2 tbsp garlic-infused olive oil, divided
- 8 oz medium shrimp, peeled and deveined
- Salt and pepper, to taste
- 1 cup bell pepper, sliced
- 1 cup zucchini, sliced
- 1/4 cup green onions (green tops only), sliced
- 2 tbsp soy sauce (gluten-free)
- 1 tbsp rice vinegar
- 1 tsp fresh ginger, grated
- 1/4 tsp red pepper flakes (optional)

Directions:

- Cook rice noodles according to package instructions, then drain and set aside.
- In a large skillet or wok, heat 1 tablespoon of garlic-infused olive oil over medium-high heat.
- Season shrimp with salt and pepper, then add to the skillet. Cook for 2-3 minutes per side or until pink and cooked through. Remove shrimp from the skillet and set aside.
- In the same skillet, add the remaining olive oil, bell pepper, and zucchini. Cook for 3-4 minutes, or until vegetables are tender-crisp.
- Stir in scallions, cooked shrimp, and cooked rice noodles.
- In a small bowl, whisk together soy sauce, rice vinegar, ginger, and red pepper flakes, if using. Pour sauce over the stir-fry and toss to combine.
- Serve immediately.

Note: In choosing rice noodles, check the ingredient's nutrition label list. Watch out for wheat or rye or barley since these ingredients have high FODMAP content.

Nutrition Information (per serving): Calories: 485, Protein: 29.9g, Fat: 16g, Carbohydrates: 56.3g, Fiber: 2.8g, Sugar: 4.3g

Day 4

Day 4 - Breakfast Banana and Almond Butter Oat Muffins

Description: A delicious and easy-to-make snack or breakfast option that's low in FODMAPs.

Preparation and Cooking Time: 35 minutes

Number of Servings: 12

Ingredients:

- 2 cups rolled oats
- 1 tsp baking powder
- 1/2 tsp cinnamon
- 1/4 tsp salt
- 2 "just ripe" bananas, mashed
- 1/2 cup almond butter
- 1/4 cup maple syrup
- 1/4 cup lactose-free milk
- 2 large eggs
- 1 tsp vanilla extract
- 1/2 cup dark chocolate chips (optional)

Directions:

- Preheat the oven to 350°F (177°C) and line a 12-cup muffin tin with paper liners.

- In a large bowl, combine the rolled oats, baking powder, cinnamon, and salt.
- In a separate bowl, mix the mashed bananas, almond butter, maple syrup, lactose-free milk or almond milk, eggs, and vanilla extract until smooth.
- Stir the wet ingredients into the dry ingredients until just combined, then fold in the dark chocolate chips, if using.
- Divide the batter evenly among the muffin cups, filling each about 3/4 full.
- Bake for 20-25 minutes, or until a toothpick inserted into the center of a muffin comes out clean. Allow the muffins to cool in the pan for 5 minutes before transferring to a wire rack to cool completely.

Substitution ideas: You can replace lactose-free milk with plant-based milk such as almond or soy milk (made from isolated soy proteins).

Nutrition Information (per serving, excluding chocolate chips): Calories: 169, Protein: 4.8g, Fat: 8.1g, Carbohydrates: 21g, Fiber: 2.3g, Sugar: 7.3g

Day 4 - Lunch: Low-FODMAP Chicken Salad Lettuce Wraps

Description: A refreshing and light lunch option featuring a flavorful chicken salad served in crisp lettuce leaves for a low-FODMAP meal.

Preparation and Cooking Time: 15 minutes

Number of Servings: 2

Ingredients:
- 1 cup cooked chicken breast, diced

- 1/4 cup red bell pepper, diced
- 1/4 cup cucumber, diced
- 2 tbsp plain mayonnaise
- 1 tbsp fresh dill, chopped
- Salt and pepper, to taste
- 4 large lettuce leaves (iceberg or butter lettuce)

Directions:

- In a medium bowl, combine the chicken, red bell pepper, cucumber, mayonnaise, and dill. Mix well and season with salt and pepper.
- Spoon the chicken salad onto the lettuce leaves and fold to create wraps.
- Serve immediately or refrigerate until ready to eat.

Nutrition Information (per serving):   Calories: 211, Protein: 21g, Fat: 12.3g, Carbohydrates: 3.4g, Fiber: 0.7g, Sugar: 1.3g

Day 4 - Dinner: Low-FODMAP Spinach-Stuffed Baked Salmon

Description: A delicious and healthy dinner option featuring tender baked salmon fillets stuffed with a flavorful spinach and feta mixture.

Preparation and Cooking Time: 40 minutes

Number of Servings: 2

Ingredients:

- 2 (6 oz each) salmon fillets
- Salt and pepper, to taste
- 1 tbsp garlic-infused olive oil
- 2 cups fresh baby spinach

- 1/4 cup feta cheese, crumbled
- 1/4 cup fresh basil, chopped
- Zest of 1 lemon

Directions:

- Preheat your oven to 375°F (190°C). Grease a baking dish and set aside.
- Season salmon fillets with salt and pepper. Using a sharp knife, cut a deep slit in the center of each fillet, creating a pocket for the stuffing.
- In a skillet, heat the garlic-infused olive oil over medium heat. Add spinach and cook until wilted, about 2-3 minutes. Remove from heat and let it cool slightly.
- In a small bowl, combine the cooked spinach, feta cheese, basil, and lemon zest. Mix well.
- Stuff each salmon fillet with the spinach mixture, then place the stuffed fillets in the prepared baking dish.
- Bake for 20-25 minutes, or until the salmon is cooked through and flakes easily with a fork.
- Serve immediately.

Nutrition Information (per serving): Calories: 389, Protein: 44.6g, Fat: 23.1g, Carbohydrates: 2g, Fiber: 0.7g, Sugar: 0.9g

Day 5

Day 5 - Breakfast: Low-FODMAP Berry Smoothie

Description: A tasty, refreshing smoothie made with low-FODMAP berries and lactose-free yogurt for a quick and easy breakfast.

Preparation and Cooking Time: 5 minutes

233

Number of Servings: 2

Ingredients:

- 1 cup lactose-free yogurt
- 1 cup frozen mixed berries (strawberries, blueberries, and raspberries)
- 1/2 cup unsweetened almond milk
- 1 tbsp chia seeds (optional)
- 1 tbsp maple syrup or low-FODMAP sweetener of choice

Directions:

- Place all ingredients in a blender and blend until smooth.
- Pour the smoothie into two glasses and enjoy immediately.

Substitution ideas: You can replace lactose-free yogurt with plant-based yogurts such as almond or soy yogurt (made from isolated soy proteins). You can also use table sugar as a low-FODMAP sweetener.

Nutrition Information (per serving): Calories: 196, Protein: 3.9g, Fat: 7.8g, Carbohydrates: 28.2g, Fiber: 6.2g, Sugar: 16g

Day 5 - Lunch: Low-FODMAP Quinoa Tabbouleh Salad

Description: A light and refreshing salad featuring quinoa, cherry tomatoes, cucumber, and a zesty lemon dressing for a low-FODMAP twist on a classic dish.

Preparation and Cooking Time: 30 minutes

Number of Servings: 4

Ingredients:

- 1 cup quinoa, uncooked
- 2 cups water
- 1 cup cherry tomatoes, halved
- 1 cup cucumber, diced
- 1/4 cup fresh parsley, chopped
- 1/4 cup fresh mint, chopped
- 2 tbsp garlic-infused olive oil
- 1 pc lemon, juiced
- Salt and pepper, to taste

Directions:

- In a medium saucepan, combine quinoa and water. Bring to a boil, then reduce heat to low, cover, and simmer for 15 minutes or until the quinoa is cooked and the water is absorbed.
- Fluff the cooked quinoa with a fork and transfer it to a large bowl. Allow it to cool completely.
- Add the cherry tomatoes, cucumber, parsley, and mint to the cooled quinoa. Toss gently to combine.
- In a small bowl, whisk together the garlic-infused olive oil and lemon juice. Season with salt and pepper.
- Pour the dressing over the quinoa salad and toss well to combine. Serve immediately or refrigerate for later.

Nutrition Information (per serving): Calories: 238, Protein: 7.1g, Fat: 9.8g, Carbohydrates: 31.7g, Fiber: 4.2g, Sugar: 2.2g

Day 5 - Dinner: Low-FODMAP Shrimp and Broccoli Stir-Fry

Description: A quick and easy dinner featuring succulent shrimp and fresh broccoli stir-fried in a flavorful, low-FODMAP sauce.

Preparation and Cooking Time: 20 minutes

Number of Servings: 4

Ingredients:

- 1 lb large shrimp, peeled and deveined
- 2 cups broccoli florets
- 1 tbsp garlic-infused olive oil
- 1/4 cup low-sodium soy sauce (gluten-free)
- 1 tbsp rice vinegar
- 1 tbsp maple syrup
- 1 tbsp cornstarch
- 2 tbsp water
- Salt and pepper, to taste

Directions:

- In a large skillet or wok, heat the garlic-infused olive oil over medium-high heat. Add the shrimp and cook until they turn pink, about 3-4 minutes. Remove the shrimp from the skillet and set aside.
- In the same skillet, add the broccoli florets and cook for 3-4 minutes, or until they're crisp-tender.
- In a small bowl, whisk together the soy sauce, rice vinegar, and maple syrup.
- In another small bowl, mix the cornstarch and water to create a slurry.
- Add the cooked shrimp back to the skillet with the broccoli. Pour the soy sauce mixture and the cornstarch slurry into the skillet, stirring continuously until the sauce thickens.
- Season with salt and pepper to taste. Serve immediately over cooked rice or low-FODMAP noodles.

Nutrition Information (per serving): Calories: 198, Protein: 26.1g, Fat: 5.5g, Carbohydrates: 11.2g, Fiber: 2g, Sugar: 5g

Day 6

Day 6 - Breakfast: Low-FODMAP Spinach and Tomato Omelet

Description: A delicious and nutritious omelette packed with spinach, tomatoes, and lactose-free cheese for a protein-rich breakfast.

Preparation and Cooking Time: 15 minutes

Number of Servings: 1

Ingredients:
- 2 large eggs
- Salt and pepper, to taste
- 1 tsp garlic-infused olive oil
- 1/2 cup fresh spinach, chopped
- 1/4 cup tomatoes, diced
- 1/4 cup grated lactose-free cheese

Directions:
- In a small bowl, whisk together the eggs with salt and pepper to taste.
- Heat the garlic-infused olive oil in a non-stick skillet over medium heat. Add the spinach and tomatoes, and cook for 2-3 minutes until the spinach is wilted.
- Pour the eggs over the spinach and tomatoes, and let them cook for a few minutes until they begin to set.
- Sprinkle the lactose-free cheese over one-half of the omelette. Fold the other half over the cheese, and let it cook for another 1-2 minutes until the cheese is melted.
- Carefully slide the omelette onto a plate and enjoy!

Substitution ideas: You can use feta, brie, camembert, or hard cheeses as your lactose-free cheese.

Nutrition Information (per serving, feta cheese used for the computation): Calories: 294, Protein: 18.8g, Fat: 22.7g, Carbohydrates: 4.7g, Fiber: 0.9g, Sugar: 3.5g

Day 6 - Lunch: Low-FODMAP Chicken and Grape Salad

Description: A delicious and refreshing salad that combines tender chicken breast, sweet grapes, and crunchy celery with a creamy, low-FODMAP dressing.

Preparation and Cooking Time: 15 minutes

Number of Servings: 4

Ingredients:
- 1 lb or 2 cups cooked chicken breast, shredded
- 1 cup red or green seedless grapes, halved
- 1/2 cup celery, diced
- 1/4 cup chives, chopped
- 1/2 cup lactose-free yogurt
- 1 tbsp Dijon mustard
- Salt and pepper, to taste

Directions:
- In a large bowl, combine the shredded chicken, grapes, celery, and chives.
- In a small bowl, whisk together the lactose-free yogurt or mayonnaise and Dijon mustard.

- Pour the dressing over the chicken mixture and toss gently to combine. Season with salt and pepper to taste.
- Serve the salad on its own, in a lettuce wrap, or on gluten-free bread for a delicious low-FODMAP sandwich.

Substitution ideas: You can replace lactose-free yogurt with plant-based yogurts such as almond or soy yogurt (made from isolated soy proteins).

Nutrition Information (per serving): Calories: 160, Protein: 21.4g, Fat: 3.5g, Carbohydrates: 10.3g, Fiber: 0.9g, Sugar: 7.6g

Day 6 - Dinner: Low-FODMAP Lemon Herb Baked Salmon

Description: A simple and flavorful dinner featuring baked salmon with a zesty lemon and herb marinade.

Preparation and Cooking Time: 30 minutes

Number of Servings: 4

Ingredients:

- 4 (6 oz each) salmon fillets
- 1/4 cup garlic-infused olive oil
- 1 pc lemon, juiced
- 1 tbsp fresh dill, chopped
- 1 tbsp fresh parsley, chopped
- Salt and pepper, to taste

Directions:

- Preheat the oven to 400°F (200°C). Line a baking sheet with parchment paper or aluminum foil.

- In a small bowl, whisk together the garlic-infused olive oil, lemon juice, dill, and parsley.
- Place the salmon fillets on the prepared baking sheet, skin side down. Pour the lemon herb mixture over the salmon fillets, making sure they're well coated.
- Season the salmon with salt and pepper to taste. Bake for 15-20 minutes or until the salmon flakes easily with a fork.
- Serve the baked salmon with a side of steamed vegetables such as green beans, bok choy, zucchini, potato, or a low-FODMAP salad for a complete, delicious meal.

Nutrition Information (per serving): Calories: 387, Protein: 41.4g, Fat: 24.7g, Carbohydrates: 1.9g, Fiber: 0.6g, Sugar: 0.4g

Day 7

Day 7 - Breakfast: Low-FODMAP Chia Pudding

Description: A simple, make-ahead chia pudding with almond milk and a hint of vanilla for a delicious and nutritious low-FODMAP breakfast.

Preparation and Cooking Time: 5 minutes (plus at least 2 hours of chilling time)

Number of Servings: 2

Ingredients:
- 1/4 cup chia seeds
- 1 cup unsweetened almond milk
- 1/2 tsp vanilla extract
- 1 tbsp maple syrup or low-FODMAP sweetener of choice

- Optional toppings: low-FODMAP fruit

Directions:

- In a medium bowl or mason jar, combine the chia seeds, almond milk, vanilla extract, and sweetener. Stir well to combine.
- Cover the mixture and refrigerate for at least 2 hours, or overnight for a thicker consistency.
- When ready to serve, give the chia pudding a good stir and divide it between two bowls or glasses. Top with your choice of low-FODMAP fruit, lactose-free yogurt, or nuts.

Substitution ideas: You can use table sugar as a low-FODMAP sweetener. In choosing low-FODMAP foods as your toppings, you may use nuts, fruits such as cantaloupe, kiwi, and berries, and lactose-free yogurt or plant-based yogurts such as almond or soy milk (made from isolated soy proteins).

Nutrition Information (per serving): Calories: 187, Protein: 5.2g, Fat: 10.5g, Carbohydrates: 19.8g, Fiber: 10.2g, Sugar: 6.1g

Day 7 - Lunch: Low-FODMAP Greek Salad

Description: A fresh, vibrant Greek salad with juicy tomatoes, crisp cucumbers, and olives, all tossed in a zesty lemon-olive oil dressing.

Preparation and Cooking Time: 15 minutes

Number of Servings: 4

Ingredients:

- 2 cups romaine lettuce, chopped
- 1 cup cherry tomatoes, halved
- 1 cup cucumber, diced

- 1/2 cup kalamata olives, pitted
- 1/2 cup red bell pepper, diced
- 1/4 cup feta cheese, crumbled
- 1/4 cup fresh parsley, chopped
- 1 1/3 pc lemon, juiced
- 1/4 cup olive oil
- Salt and pepper, to taste

Directions:
- Combine the romaine lettuce, cherry tomatoes, cucumber, kalamata olives, red bell pepper, and feta cheese in a large salad bowl.
- In a small bowl, whisk together the lemon juice, olive oil, salt, and pepper. Pour the dressing over the salad and toss well to combine.
- Garnish the salad with chopped fresh parsley and serve immediately.

Nutrition Information (per serving): Calories: 183, Protein: 3.7g, Fat: 16.8g, Carbohydrates: 6.8g, Fiber: 1.8g, Sugar: 3g

Day 7 - Dinner: Low-FODMAP Spaghetti Squash with Pesto

Description: A delicious, low-FODMAP alternative to pasta using spaghetti squash and homemade basil pesto.

Preparation and Cooking Time: 60 minutes

Number of Servings: 4

Ingredients:
- 1 (about 3 lb) medium spaghetti squash
- 1 tbsp olive oil

- Salt and pepper, to taste

For Pesto:

- 2 cups fresh basil leaves
- 1/3 cup pine nuts
- 1/3 cup Parmesan cheese, grated
- 1/2 cup olive oil
- 1/3 pc of lemon, juiced
- 1/4 tsp salt

Directions:

- Preheat your oven to 400°F (200°C). Cut the spaghetti squash in half lengthwise and remove the seeds. Drizzle the cut sides with olive oil and season with salt and pepper. Place the squash halves cut-side down on a baking sheet and roast for 40-45 minutes, or until the squash is tender and easily pierced with a fork.
- While the squash is roasting, prepare the pesto. In a food processor, combine the basil, pine nuts, Parmesan cheese, olive oil, lemon juice, and salt. Process until smooth, scraping down the sides as needed.
- Once the squash is cooked, let it cool slightly before using a fork to scrape the flesh into spaghetti-like strands. Transfer the spaghetti squash strands to a serving bowl.
- Toss the spaghetti squash with the pesto, ensuring it is well coated. Serve immediately.

Nutrition Information (per serving): Calories: 449, Protein: 11.1g, Fat: 44.2g, Carbohydrates: 9.2g, Fiber: 2.8g, Sugar: 4.8g

Day 8

Day 8 - Breakfast: Low-FODMAP Berry Smoothie

Description: A refreshing and nutritious berry smoothie made with lactose-free yogurt and a mix of your favorite low-FODMAP berries.

Preparation and Cooking Time: 5 minutes

Number of Servings: 1

Ingredients:
- 1 cup lactose-free yogurt (plain or vanilla)
- 1/2 cup frozen mixed low-FODMAP berries
- 1 tbsp chia seeds
- 1 tbsp maple syrup or low-FODMAP sweetener of choice (optional)

Directions:
- In a blender, combine the lactose-free yogurt, frozen mixed berries, chia seeds, and maple syrup or sweetener (if using).
- Blend until smooth and creamy.
- Pour the smoothie into a glass and serve immediately.

Substitution ideas: You can replace lactose-free milk with plant-based milk such as almond or soy milk (made from isolated soy proteins). When choosing low-FODMAP berries, start with strawberries, blueberries, and raspberries. You can use table sugar as a low-FODMAP sweetener.

Nutrition Information (per serving): Calories: 311, Protein: 11.3g, Fat: 12.6g, Carbohydrates: 39.3g, Fiber: 7.4g, Sugar: 28.3g

Day 8 - Lunch: Low-FODMAP Tuna Salad Lettuce Wraps

Description: Light and tasty lettuce wraps filled with a flavorful tuna salad made with low-FODMAP ingredients.

Preparation and Cooking Time: 15 minutes

Number of Servings: 2

Ingredients:

- 1 (5 oz) can of tuna in water, drained
- 1/4 cup cucumber, diced
- 1/4 cup red bell pepper, diced
- 1/4 cup plain mayonnaise
- 1 tbsp Dijon mustard
- 1 tbsp fresh dill, chopped
- Salt and pepper, to taste
- 4 large lettuce leaves (Iceberg Lettuce or Butter lettuce)

Directions:

- In a medium bowl, mix the tuna, cucumber, red bell pepper, mayonnaise, Dijon mustard, and fresh dill. Season with salt and pepper, to taste.
- Lay the lettuce leaves on a flat surface and spoon the tuna salad evenly onto each leaf.
- Carefully fold or roll the lettuce leaves around the tuna salad, tucking in the edges as you go. Serve immediately.

Nutrition Information (per serving): Calories: 309, Protein: 17.7g, Fat: 24.6g, Carbohydrates: 3.4g, Fiber: 0.9g, Sugar: 1.2g

Day 8 - Dinner: Low-FODMAP Chicken Stir-Fry

Description: A flavorful and satisfying chicken stir-fry with colorful veggies and a savory low-FODMAP sauce.

Preparation and Cooking Time: 30 minutes

Number of Servings: 4

Ingredients:

- 1 lb boneless, skinless chicken breasts, thinly sliced
- 2 tbsp olive oil, divided
- 1 cup bell peppers (any color), chopped
- 1 cup zucchini, chopped
- 1/2 cup green onions (green tops only), chopped
- 1/4 cup low-sodium soy sauce or tamari (gluten-free)
- 1 tbsp maple syrup
- 1 tbsp cornstarch
- Salt and pepper, to taste

Directions:

- Heat 1 tablespoon of olive oil in a large skillet or wok over medium-high heat. Add the sliced chicken and cook until browned and cooked through, about 4-5 minutes per side. Transfer the chicken to a plate and set aside.
- In the same skillet, heat the remaining tablespoon of olive oil. Add the bell peppers, zucchini, and green onion tops. Cook the vegetables, stirring occasionally, until they are tender-crisp, about 5 minutes.
- In a small bowl, whisk together the soy sauce, maple syrup, and cornstarch until smooth. Pour the sauce mixture over the vegetables in the skillet and cook for an additional 2-3 minutes, or until the sauce has thickened.
- Return the cooked chicken to the skillet and stir to combine with the vegetables and sauce. Cook for another 2 minutes, or

until everything is heated through. Season with salt and pepper, to taste.

- Serve the chicken stir-fry over cooked rice or low-FODMAP noodles, if desired.

Nutrition Information (per serving): Calories: 319, Protein: 34.7g, Fat: 15.6g, Carbohydrates: 10.3g, Fiber: 1.1g, Sugar: 6.3g

Day 9

Day 9 - Breakfast: Low-FODMAP Veggie Omelette

Description: A filling and nutritious omelette loaded with low-FODMAP veggies and cheese.

Preparation and Cooking Time: 15 minutes

Number of Servings: 1 Serving Size: 1 omelette

Ingredients:
- 2 large eggs
- 2 tbsp lactose-free milk
- Salt and pepper, to taste
- 1 tbsp olive oil
- 1/4 cup chopped bell peppers
- 1/4 cup chopped tomatoes
- 2 tbsp chopped chives
- 1/4 cup grated cheddar cheese

Directions:
- In a bowl, whisk together the eggs, milk, salt, and pepper.

- Heat the olive oil in a non-stick skillet over medium heat. Add the bell peppers and cook for 2-3 minutes until softened.
- Add the tomatoes and cook for another 1-2 minutes.
- Pour the egg mixture into the skillet and cook until almost set, lifting the edges to allow the uncooked eggs to flow underneath.
- Sprinkle the cheese and chives on one half of the omelette. Fold the other half over the filling and cook for another 1-2 minutes until the cheese is melted.

Substitution ideas: You can replace lactose-free milk with plant-based milk such as almond or soy milk (made from isolated soy proteins).

Nutrition Information (per serving): Calories: 413, Protein: 21.5g, Fat: 34.1g, Carbohydrates: 7.1g, Fiber: 1.1g, Sugar: 5.2g

Day 9 - Lunch: Low-FODMAP Greek Salad with Chicken

Description: A refreshing and protein-packed Greek salad topped with grilled chicken for a satisfying lunch.

Preparation and Cooking Time: 25 minutes

Number of Servings: 4

Ingredients:
- 1 lb boneless, skinless chicken breasts
- 1 tbsp olive oil
- Salt and pepper, to taste
- 6 cups lettuce (Romaine or iceberg lettuce), chopped
- 1 cup cherry tomatoes, halved
- 1 cup cucumber, chopped
- 1/4 cup kalamata olives, pitted and sliced

- 1/4 cup crumbled feta cheese (optional)
- 1/4 cup low-FODMAP Greek salad dressing

Directions:

- Preheat a grill or grill pan to medium heat. Rub the chicken breasts with olive oil and season with salt and pepper. Grill the chicken for 5-7 minutes per side, or until cooked through and the internal temperature reaches 165°F (75°C). Let the chicken rest for a few minutes before slicing.
- In a large bowl, combine the lettuce, cherry tomatoes, cucumber, and olives. Toss with the low-FODMAP Greek salad dressing.
- Divide the salad among four plates or bowls. Top each serving with sliced grilled chicken and crumbled feta cheese, if using.

In choosing a low-FODMAP Greek salad dressing, check the ingredient's nutrition label list. Watch out for onion or garlic since these ingredients have high FODMAP content.

Nutrition Information (per serving, excluding the feta cheese): Calories: 345, Protein: 34.2g, Fat: 20.8g, Carbohydrates: 6.4g, Fiber: 1.2g, Sugar: 3.4g

Day 9 - Dinner: Low-FODMAP Shrimp and Vegetable Stir-Fry

Description: A quick and flavorful shrimp stir-fry with colorful veggies and a savory low-FODMAP sauce.

Preparation and Cooking Time: 30 minutes

Number of Servings: 4

Ingredients:

- 1 lb large shrimp, peeled and deveined
- 2 tbsp olive oil, divided
- 1 cup bell peppers (any color), chopped
- 1 cup zucchini, chopped
- 1/2 cup green onions (green tops only), chopped
- 1/4 cup low-sodium soy sauce or tamari (gluten-free)
- 1 tbsp maple syrup
- 1 tbsp cornstarch
- Salt and pepper, to taste

Directions:

- Heat 1 tablespoon of olive oil in a large skillet or wok over medium-high heat. Add the shrimp and cook until pink and cooked through, about 2-3 minutes per side. Transfer the shrimp to a plate and set aside.
- In the same skillet, heat the remaining tablespoon of olive oil. Add the bell peppers, zucchini, and green onion tops. Cook the vegetables, stirring occasionally, until they are tender-crisp, about 5 minutes.
- In a small bowl, whisk together the soy sauce, maple syrup, and cornstarch until smooth. Pour the sauce mixture over the vegetables in the skillet and cook for an additional 2-3 minutes, or until the sauce has thickened.
- Return the cooked shrimp to the skillet and stir to combine with the vegetables and sauce. Cook for another 2 minutes, or until everything is heated through. Season with salt and pepper, to taste.
- Serve the shrimp stir-fry over cooked rice or low-FODMAP noodles, if desired.

Nutrition Information (per serving): Calories: 255, Protein: 32.1g, Fat: 9.9g, Carbohydrates: 10.3g, Fiber: 1.1g, Sugar: 6.3g

Day 10

Day 10 - Breakfast Quinoa with Blueberries and Pecans

Description: A high-protein, gluten-free alternative to oatmeal that's packed with antioxidants.

Preparation and Cooking Time: 25 minutes

Number of Servings: 4

Ingredients:

- 1 cup quinoa, uncooked, rinsed, and drained
- 2 cups water
- 1/4 tsp salt
- 1 cup blueberries
- 1/2 cup chopped pecans
- 1/4 cup maple syrup
- 1 cup lactose-free yogurt

Directions:

- In a medium saucepan, combine the quinoa, water, and salt. Bring to a boil, then reduce heat to low and simmer for 15 minutes, or until the quinoa is tender and the water is absorbed.
- Remove from heat and let the quinoa sit, covered, for 5 minutes.
- Fluff the quinoa with a fork, then divide it among four bowls.
- Top each serving with blueberries, pecans, maple syrup, and lactose-free yogurt or almond milk.

Substitution ideas: You can replace lactose-free yogurt with plant-based yogurts such as almond or soy yogurt (made from isolated soy proteins).

Nutrition Information (per serving): Calories: 292, Protein: 8.8g, Fat: 7.5g, Carbohydrates: 49.1g, Fiber: 4.2g, Sugar: 18.3g

Day 10 - Lunch: Low-FODMAP Greek Salad

Description: A refreshing and flavorful Greek salad filled with crunchy vegetables, olives, and feta cheese.

Preparation Time: 15 minutes

Number of Servings: 4

Ingredients:

- 4 cups chopped lettuce (romaine or iceberg lettuce)
- 1 large cucumber, peeled and chopped
- 1 cup cherry tomatoes, halved
- 1/2 cup Kalamata olives, pitted & halved
- 1/2 cup feta cheese, crumbled
- 1/4 cup green onions (green tops only), chopped
- 1/4 cup fresh parsley, chopped
- 1/4 cup olive oil
- 2 tbsp red wine vinegar
- 1/2 tsp dried oregano
- Salt and pepper, to taste

Directions:

- Combine the lettuce, cucumber, cherry tomatoes, olives, feta cheese, green onion tops, and parsley in a large salad bowl.

- In a small bowl, whisk together the olive oil, red wine vinegar, dried oregano, salt, and pepper.
- Drizzle the dressing over the salad and toss to combine. Serve immediately.

Nutrition Information (per serving): Calories: 209, Protein: 4.2g, Fat: 18.7g, Carbohydrates: 8.9g, Fiber: 2.2g, Sugar: 4g

Day 10 - Dinner: Low-FODMAP Shrimp and Vegetable Stir-Fry

Description: A quick and delicious shrimp and vegetable stir-fry with a flavorful garlic and ginger sauce.

Preparation and Cooking Time: 30 minutes

Number of Servings: 4

Ingredients:
- 1 lb shrimp, peeled and deveined
- 1 cup bell peppers (red, yellow, or orange), chopped
- 1 cup zucchini, chopped
- 1 cup carrots, chopped
- 1/4 cup green onions (green tops only), chopped
- 2 tbsp garlic-infused olive oil, divided
- 1 tbsp fresh ginger, grated
- 3 tbsp low-sodium soy sauce or tamari (gluten-free)
- 1 tbsp rice vinegar
- 1 tbsp cornstarch
- 1/4 cup water
- Salt and pepper, to taste

Directions:

- In a large skillet or wok, heat 1 tablespoon of garlic-infused olive oil over medium-high heat. Add the shrimp and cook until pink and cooked through, about 2-3 minutes per side. Remove the shrimp from the skillet and set aside.
- Add the remaining tablespoon of olive oil to the skillet. Add the bell peppers, zucchini, carrots, and green onion tops. Cook, stirring frequently, until the vegetables are tender-crisp, about 5 minutes.
- In a small bowl, whisk together the ginger, soy sauce, rice vinegar, cornstarch, and water. Pour the sauce over the vegetables and cook, stirring, until the sauce thickens about 2 minutes.
- Add the cooked shrimp back to the skillet and cook until heated through, about 1 minute. Season with salt and pepper to taste.
- Serve the stir-fry over cooked rice or quinoa, if desired.

Nutrition Information (per serving): Calories: 241, Protein: 27.7g, Fat: 9.1g, Carbohydrates: 11.6g, Fiber: 1.8g, Sugar: 4.3g

Day 11

Day 11 - Breakfast: Low-FODMAP Blueberry Smoothie

Description: A creamy and refreshing blueberry smoothie, perfect for a quick and easy low-FODMAP breakfast.

Preparation Time: 5 minutes

Number of Servings: 2

Ingredients:
- 1 cup frozen blueberries
- 1 cup lactose-free yogurt
- 1 cup lactose-free milk
- 1 tbsp chia seeds
- 1 tbsp maple syrup or low FODMAP sweetener

Directions:
- In a blender, combine the frozen blueberries, yogurt, milk, chia seeds, and sweetener (if using).
- Blend on high speed until smooth and creamy. Pour the smoothie into two glasses and serve immediately.

Substitution ideas: You can replace lactose-free yogurt/milk with plant-based yogurt/milk such as coconut, almond, or soy yogurt/milk (made from isolated soy proteins). You can use table sugar as a low-FODMAP sweetener.

Nutrition Information (per serving): Calories: 242, Protein: 10g, Fat: 8.9g, Carbohydrates: 32.4g, Fiber: 4.2g, Sugar: 24.9g

Day 11 - Lunch: Low-FODMAP Chicken Caesar Salad

Description: A classic Caesar salad made low-FODMAP with a home-made dressing and grilled chicken.

Preparation and Cooking Time: 30 minutes

Number of Servings: 4

Ingredients:

- 4 cups romaine lettuce, chopped
- 1 lb boneless, skinless chicken breasts
- Salt and pepper, to taste
- 1/2 cup Parmesan cheese, grated
- 1 cup gluten-free croutons

Dressing:

- 1/2 cup lactose-free sour cream
- 1/4 cup Parmesan cheese, grated
- 1/3 pc lemon, juiced
- 1 tbsp garlic-infused olive oil
- 1 tbsp anchovy paste (optional)
- 1 tsp Dijon mustard
- Salt and pepper, to taste

Directions:

- Preheat a grill or grill pan to medium-high heat. Season the chicken breasts with salt and pepper, then grill for 6-7 minutes per side, or until cooked through and the internal temperature reaches 165°F (74°C). Remove the chicken from the grill and let it rest for a few minutes before slicing.
- In a small bowl, whisk together the dressing ingredients until smooth. Taste and adjust seasoning as needed.
- In a large bowl, combine the chopped romaine lettuce, sliced grilled chicken, Parmesan cheese, and gluten-free croutons. Drizzle the dressing over the salad and toss to combine.
- Divide the salad among four plates and serve.

Nutrition Information (per serving excluding anchovy paste): Calories: 373, Protein: 40.2g, Fat: 17.6g, Carbohydrates: 10.2g, Fiber: 0.8g, Sugar: 3.5g

Day 11 - Dinner: Low-FODMAP Veggie-Packed Bolognese

Description: A comforting and flavorful Bolognese sauce packed with vegetables and served over gluten-free pasta.

Preparation and Cooking Time: 60 minutes

Number of Servings: 6

Ingredients:

- 1 lb lean ground beef
- 1 cup carrots, chopped
- 1 cup zucchini, chopped
- 1 cup red bell pepper, chopped
- 1/4 cup green onions (green tops only), chopped
- 2 tbsp garlic-infused olive oil
- 1 (28 oz) can of crushed tomatoes
- 1 tbsp dried basil
- 1 tbsp dried oregano
- Salt and pepper, to taste
- 12 oz gluten-free spaghetti or pasta of choice, cooked according to package directions

Directions:

- In a large skillet, heat the garlic-infused olive oil over medium heat. Add the ground meat and cook, breaking it up with a spoon, until browned and cooked through about 10 minutes. Remove the meat from the skillet and set aside.
- In the same skillet, add the carrots, zucchini, bell pepper, and green onion tops. Cook, stirring occasionally, until the vegetables are tender, about 10 minutes.
- Add the cooked meat back to the skillet, along with the crushed tomatoes, basil, and oregano. Stir well to combine. Bring the sauce to a simmer, then reduce the heat to low and cook, cov-

ered, for 20 minutes, stirring occasionally. Season the sauce with salt and pepper to taste.

- Serve the Bolognese sauce over cooked gluten-free pasta.

Nutrition Information (per serving): Calories: 472, Protein: 33.1g, Fat: 11.1g, Carbohydrates: 57.9g, Fiber: 8.7g, Sugar: 10.4g

Day 12

Day 12 - Breakfast: Low-FODMAP Banana Pancakes

Description: Start your day with these fluffy, delicious banana pancakes that are low in FODMAPs and easy to make.

Preparation and Cooking Time: 20 minutes

Number of Servings: 4

Ingredients:
- 1 cup gluten-free all-purpose flour
- 1 tbsp granulated sugar
- 1/2 tsp baking powder
- 1/2 tsp baking soda
- 1/4 tsp salt
- 1 cup lactose-free milk
- 1 large egg
- 1 tbsp vegetable oil
- 1 "just ripe" banana
- Cooking spray for the pan

Directions:

- In a large bowl, whisk together the gluten-free flour, sugar, baking powder, baking soda, and salt.
- Whisk together the lactose-free milk, egg, and vegetable oil in a separate bowl. Stir in the mashed banana.
- Pour the wet ingredients into the dry ingredients and stir until just combined. Do not overmix.
- Heat a large nonstick skillet or griddle over medium heat and lightly coat with cooking spray.
- Pour 1/4 cup of the pancake batter onto the hot skillet for each pancake. Cook for 2-3 minutes, or until bubbles form on the surface and the edges look set. Flip the pancakes and cook for an additional 1-2 minutes or until golden brown and cooked through.
- Serve the pancakes with your choice of low-FODMAP toppings, such as maple syrup or fresh berries.

Substitution ideas: You can use rice flour, or potato starch as your gluten-free flour. You can replace lactose-free milk with plant-based milk such as almond or soy milk (made from isolated soy proteins).

Nutrition Information (per serving): Calories: 225, Protein: 6.9g, Fat: 6.7g, Carbohydrates: 35.4g, Fiber: 3.8g, Sugar: 9.7g

Day 12 - Lunch: Low-FODMAP Greek Salad

Description: A refreshing and flavorful Greek salad that's perfect for a light and healthy lunch.

Preparation and Cooking Time: 15 minutes

Number of Servings: 4

Ingredients:

- 1 large cucumber, peeled and chopped
- 1/2 cup cherry tomatoes, halved
- 1/2 cup Kalamata olives, pitted & halved
- 1/2 cup feta cheese, crumbled
- 1/4 cup green onions (green tops only), chopped
- 2 tbsp fresh parsley, chopped
- 1/4 cup extra-virgin olive oil
- 2 tbsp red wine vinegar
- 1/2 tsp dried oregano
- Salt and pepper, to taste

Directions:

- In a large bowl, combine the cucumber, cherry tomatoes, olives, feta cheese, green onion tops, and parsley.
- In a small bowl, whisk together the olive oil, red wine vinegar, oregano, salt, and pepper.
- Pour the dressing over the salad and toss to combine. Let the salad sit for a few minutes to allow the flavors to meld, then serve.

Nutrition Information (per serving): Calories: 197, Protein: 3.7g, Fat: 18.6g, Carbohydrates: 6.2g, Fiber: 1.5g, Sugar: 2.8g

Day 12 - Dinner: Low-FODMAP Baked Lemon Herb Chicken

Description: A simple and flavorful baked chicken dish with a zesty lemon herb marinade.

Preparation and Cooking Time: 60 minutes

Number of Servings: 4

Ingredients:

- 1 lb or 4 boneless, skinless chicken breasts
- 1 1/3 pc lemon, juiced
- 1/4 cup garlic-infused olive oil
- 1 tbsp fresh parsley, chopped
- 1 tbsp fresh thyme, chopped
- Salt and pepper, to taste

Directions:

- Preheat your oven to 375°F (190°C).
- In a small bowl, whisk together the lemon juice, garlic-infused olive oil, parsley, thyme, salt, and pepper to create the marinade.
- Place the chicken breasts in a baking dish and pour the marinade over them. Make sure the chicken is fully coated in the marinade.
- Cover the baking dish with aluminum foil and bake for 25 minutes. After that, remove the foil and continue baking for an additional 10-15 minutes, or until the chicken is fully cooked and the internal temperature reaches 165°F (74°C).
- Remove the chicken from the oven and let it rest for a few minutes before serving. Spoon the pan juices over the chicken for added flavor.

Nutrition Information (per serving): Calories: 230, Protein: 26.1g, Fat: 14.2g, Carbohydrates: 0.5g, Fiber: 0.3g, Sugar: 0g

Day 13

Day 13 - Breakfast: Low-FODMAP Fruit and Nut Granola

Description: Start your day with this delicious, homemade low-FOD-MAP granola packed with nuts and dried fruits.

Preparation and Cooking Time: 60 minutes

Number of Servings: 8

Ingredients:

- 3 cups gluten-free rolled oats
- 1/2 cup walnuts, chopped
- 1/2 cup pecans, chopped
- 1/2 cup slivered almonds
- 1/2 cup unsweetened shredded coconut
- 1/4 cup chia seeds
- 1/4 cup maple syrup
- 1/4 cup melted coconut oil
- 1/2 tsp vanilla extract
- 1/2 cup dried cranberries

Directions:

- Preheat your oven to 325°F (163°C) and line a large baking sheet with parchment paper.
- In a large bowl, combine the rolled oats, walnuts, pecans, almonds, shredded coconut, and chia seeds.
- In a separate bowl, whisk together the maple syrup, melted coconut oil, and vanilla extract.
- Pour the wet ingredients over the dry ingredients and stir until everything is well coated.

- Spread the granola mixture evenly onto the prepared baking sheet.
- Bake for 30-35 minutes, stirring occasionally, until the granola is golden brown and crispy. Let the granola cool completely on the baking sheet.
- Once cooled, stir in the dried cranberries.
- Store the granola in an airtight container and serve with lactose-free yogurt or milk.

Nutrition Information (per serving): Calories: 333, Protein: 7.6g, Fat: 23.3g, Carbohydrates: 26g, Fiber: 7g, Sugar: 7g

Day 13 - Lunch: Low-FODMAP Quinoa and Roasted Veggie Salad

Description: A hearty and satisfying salad filled with roasted vegetables and protein-packed quinoa.

Preparation and Cooking Time: 60 minutes

Number of Servings: 4

Ingredients:

- 1 cup quinoa, uncooked
- 2 cups water
- 1 medium zucchini, chopped
- 1 medium bell pepper, chopped
- 1 cup cherry tomatoes, halved
- 2 tbsp garlic-infused olive oil
- Salt and pepper, to taste
- 1/4 cup chopped fresh parsley

For the dressing:

- 2/3 pc lemon, juiced
- 2 tbsp extra-virgin olive oil
- Salt and pepper, to taste

Directions:

- Preheat your oven to 425°F (218°C) and line a baking sheet with parchment paper.
- In a saucepan, combine the quinoa and water. Bring to a boil, then reduce the heat to low and cover. Cook for 15-20 minutes or until the quinoa is tender and the water is absorbed. Fluff the quinoa with a fork and set aside to cool.
- In a large bowl, toss the zucchini, bell pepper, and cherry tomatoes with the garlic-infused olive oil, salt, and pepper. Spread the vegetables in a single layer on the prepared baking sheet.
- Roast the vegetables for 20-25 minutes, or until they are tender and lightly browned. Remove them from the oven and let them cool slightly.
- In a large bowl, combine the cooked quinoa, roasted vegetables, and parsley.
- In a separate small bowl, whisk together the lemon juice and extra-virgin olive oil. Pour the dressing over the salad and toss to combine. Season with salt and pepper to taste.
- Serve the salad warm or chilled.

Nutrition Information (per serving): Calories: 305, Protein: 7.5g, Fat: 16.9g, Carbohydrates: 33.3g, Fiber: 4.6g, Sugar: 3.7g

Day 13 - Dinner: Low-FODMAP Lemon Garlic Shrimp with Zucchini Noodles

Description: A light and flavorful dinner featuring zesty lemon garlic shrimp served over a bed of spiralized zucchini noodles.

Preparation and Cooking Time: 30 minutes

Number of Servings: 4

Ingredients:

- 1 lb large shrimp, peeled and deveined
- 1/4 cup garlic-infused olive oil, divided
- 1 1/3 pc lemon, juiced
- 1/4 cup fresh parsley, chopped
- Salt and pepper, to taste
- 4 medium zucchini, spiralized into noodles
- Salt and pepper, to taste
- 1 tbsp fresh basil, chopped

Directions:

- In a large bowl, combine the shrimp, 2 tablespoons of garlic-infused olive oil, lemon juice, parsley, salt, and pepper. Toss to coat the shrimp and let them marinate for 15 minutes.
- While the shrimp marinate, heat the remaining 2 tablespoons of garlic-infused olive oil in a large skillet over medium heat. Add the spiralized zucchini noodles and cook for 3-4 minutes, or until they are tender but still retain some crunch. Season with salt and pepper to taste, then transfer the zucchini noodles to a serving platter.
- In the same skillet, cook the marinated shrimp over medium heat for 2-3 minutes per side, or until they are pink and cooked through.
- Serve the shrimp over the zucchini noodles, and garnish with chopped fresh basil.

Nutrition Information (per serving): Calories: 265, Protein: 25.7g, Fat: 15.1g, Carbohydrates: 7.2g, Fiber: 2.4g, Sugar: 3.7g

Day 14

Day 14 - Breakfast: Low-FODMAP Banana Pancakes

Description: Fluffy and delicious banana pancakes that are low-FOD-MAP and perfect for a leisurely weekend breakfast.

Preparation and Cooking Time: 25 minutes

Number of Servings: 4

Ingredients:

- 1 cup gluten-free all-purpose flour
- 1 tbsp granulated sugar
- 2 tsp baking powder
- 1/4 tsp salt
- 1 "just ripe" banana, mashed
- 1 cup lactose-free milk
- 1 large egg
- 1 tbsp vegetable oil

Directions:

- In a large bowl, whisk together the flour, sugar, baking powder, and salt. In a separate bowl, mix the mashed banana, milk, egg, and vegetable oil. Add the wet ingredients to the dry ingredients and stir until just combined.
- Preheat a non-stick griddle or large skillet over medium heat. Lightly grease it with vegetable oil. Pour about 1/4 cup of batter

for each pancake onto the griddle, and cook for about 1 minute or until bubbles form on the surface and the edges look set. Flip the pancakes and cook for another 1-2 minutes or until golden brown.

- Serve the pancakes warm with your choice of low-FODMAP toppings, such as maple syrup or fresh berries.

Substitution ideas: You can use rice flour, or potato starch as your gluten-free flour. You can replace lactose-free milk with plant-based milk such as almond or soy milk (made from isolated soy proteins).

Nutrition Information (per serving): Calories: 225, Protein: 6.9g, Fat: 6.6g, Carbohydrates: 36.3g, Fiber: 3.8g, Sugar: 9.7g

Day 14 - Lunch: Low-FODMAP Greek Salad with Grilled Chicken

Description: A refreshing and satisfying Greek salad with grilled chicken breast, cucumber, tomatoes, olives, and a tangy lemon dressing.

Preparation and Cooking Time: 30 minutes

Number of Servings: 4

Ingredients:
- 1 lb or 4 boneless, skinless chicken breasts
- 1 tbsp garlic-infused olive oil
- Salt and pepper, to taste
- 4 cups romaine lettuce, chopped
- 1 cup cherry tomatoes, halved
- 1 cup cucumber, chopped
- 1/2 cup kalamata olives, pitted & halved

- 1/4 cup feta cheese, crumbled
- 1 1/3 pc lemon, juiced
- 1/4 cup extra-virgin olive oil
- 1 tsp dried oregano

Directions:

- Preheat a grill or grill pan over medium-high heat. Brush the chicken breasts with garlic-infused olive oil, and season with salt and pepper.
- Grill the chicken for 6-8 minutes per side, or until fully cooked and the internal temperature reaches 165°F (74°C). Let the chicken rest for a few minutes, then slice it into strips.
- In a large bowl, combine the romaine lettuce, cherry tomatoes, cucumber, olives, and feta cheese (if using). In a separate small bowl, whisk together the lemon juice, extra-virgin olive oil, and oregano. Pour the dressing over the salad and toss to combine.
- Divide the salad among four plates, and top each with grilled chicken strips.

Nutrition Information (per serving): Calories: 398, Protein: 41.4g, Fat: 23.9g, Carbohydrates: 6.4g, Fiber: 1.8g, Sugar: 2.9g

Day 14 - Dinner: Low-FODMAP Shrimp and Vegetable Stir-Fry

Number of Servings: 4

Ingredients:

- 1 lb peeled and deveined shrimp
- 1 tbsp garlic-infused olive oil
- 1 cup bell peppers (any color), chopped
- 1 cup zucchini, chopped
- 1 cup carrots, chopped

- 1/4 cup low-sodium soy sauce (gluten-free)
- 1 tbsp rice vinegar
- 1 tbsp cornstarch
- 1/4 cup water
- 1 tbsp sesame oil
- 2 cups cooked brown rice (cooked according to package instructions)

Directions:

- Heat the garlic-infused olive oil in a large skillet or wok over medium-high heat. Add the shrimp and cook for 3-4 minutes, or until pink and cooked through. Remove the shrimp from the skillet and set aside.
- Add the bell peppers, zucchini, and carrots to the skillet. Stir-fry for about 5 minutes, or until the vegetables are tender-crisp.
- In a small bowl, whisk together the soy sauce or tamari, rice vinegar, cornstarch, and water to create a sauce. Pour the sauce over the vegetables in the skillet, and cook for 1-2 minutes, or until the sauce thickens.
- Add the cooked shrimp and sesame oil to the skillet, and stir to combine.
- Serve the shrimp and vegetable stir-fry over cooked rice.

Nutrition Information (per serving): Calories: 288, Protein: 29.3g, Fat: 8.7g, Carbohydrates: 24.7g, Fiber: 1.9g, Sugar: 4.3g

Day 15

Day 15 - Breakfast: Low-FODMAP Blueberry Chia Seed Pudding

Description: A creamy and delicious chia seed pudding with blueberries, perfect for a grab-and-go breakfast.

Preparation and Cooking Time: 5 minutes (plus overnight refrigeration)

Number of Servings: 2

Ingredients:
- 1 cup lactose-free milk
- 1/4 cup chia seeds
- 1 tbsp maple syrup
- 1 tsp vanilla extract
- 1/2 cup fresh blueberries

Directions:
- In a medium bowl, whisk together the milk, chia seeds, maple syrup, and vanilla extract.
- Cover the bowl and refrigerate overnight, or for at least 6 hours, until the chia seeds have absorbed the liquid and formed a pudding-like consistency.
- When ready to serve, stir the pudding well and divide it into two bowls or jars. Top with fresh blueberries.

Substitution ideas: You can replace lactose-free milk with plant-based milk such as almond or soy milk (made from isolated soy proteins).

Nutrition Information (per serving): Calories: 256, Protein: 9g, Fat: 11.4g, Carbohydrates: 30.7g, Fiber: 10.6g, Sugar: 15.8g

Day 15 - Lunch: Low-FODMAP Greek Salad with Grilled Chicken

Description: A light and refreshing Greek salad with grilled chicken, perfect for a healthy lunch option.

Preparation and Cooking Time: 30 minutes

Number of Servings: 2

Ingredients:

- ½ lb or 2 boneless, skinless chicken breasts
- 1 tbsp olive oil
- Salt and pepper, to taste
- 4 cups chopped romaine lettuce
- 1 cup cherry tomatoes, halved
- 1/2 cup chopped cucumber
- 1/4 cup pitted Kalamata olives
- 1/4 cup crumbled feta cheese

For the dressing:

- 2/3 pc lemon, juiced
- 1/4 cup extra-virgin olive oil
- 1/2 tsp dried oregano
- 1/2 tsp Dijon mustard
- Salt and pepper, to taste

Directions:

- Preheat the grill or grill pan to medium-high heat. Brush chicken breasts with olive oil and season with salt and pepper.
- Grill the chicken for 6-8 minutes per side, or until cooked through and the internal temperature reaches 165°F (75°C). Remove from grill and let rest for a few minutes before slicing.
- In a large bowl, combine the chopped lettuce, cherry tomatoes, cucumber, olives, and feta cheese.

- In a small bowl or jar, whisk together the lemon juice, extra-virgin olive oil, dried oregano, Dijon mustard, salt, and pepper to make the dressing.
- Divide the salad mixture between two plates, top with sliced grilled chicken, and drizzle with dressing.

Nutrition Information (per serving): Calories: 530, Protein: 30.5g, Fat: 42.9g, Carbohydrates: 10.2g, Fiber: 2.7g, Sugar: 5g

Day 15 - Dinner: Low-FODMAP Spaghetti Squash with Meat Sauce

Description: A delicious low-FODMAP alternative to traditional spaghetti, made with spaghetti squash and a flavorful meat sauce.

Preparation and Cooking Time: 50 minutes

Number of Servings: 4

Ingredients:

- 1 medium spaghetti squash
- 1 tbsp olive oil
- 1 lb lean ground beef
- 1 cup red bell pepper, chopped
- 1 cup zucchini, chopped
- 1/4 cup green onions (green tops only), chopped
- 2 cups low-FODMAP marinara sauce
- Salt and pepper, to taste
- 1/4 cup Parmesan cheese, grated

Directions:

- Preheat oven to 400°F (200°C). Cut the spaghetti squash in half lengthwise and scoop out the seeds.

- Place the squash halves cut-side down on a baking sheet lined with parchment paper. Bake for 35-40 minutes or until tender. Allow to cool slightly before using a fork to scrape out the spaghetti-like strands.
- While the squash is baking, heat olive oil in a large skillet over medium heat. Add the ground beef or turkey and cook, breaking it up with a spoon, until browned and cooked through about 10 minutes.
- Stir in the red bell pepper, zucchini, and green onion tops, and cook for 5-7 minutes, or until vegetables are tender.
- Add the low-FODMAP marinara sauce to the skillet, and season with salt and pepper to taste. Simmer for 10 minutes to let the flavors meld together.
- Serve the spaghetti squash topped with the meat sauce and a sprinkle of Parmesan cheese.

Note: In choosing LOW FODMAP marinara sauce, check the ingredient's nutrition label list. Watch out for onion or garlic since these ingredients have high FODMAP content.

Nutrition Information (per serving): Calories: 449, Protein: 42.4g, Fat: 18g, Carbohydrates: 29.1g, Fiber: 4.2g, Sugar: 13.8g

Day 16

Day 16 - Breakfast: Low-FODMAP Berry Smoothie Bowl

Description: A refreshing and fruity smoothie bowl packed with low-FODMAP berries and topped with crunchy granola.

Preparation and Cooking Time: 10 minutes

Number of Servings: 1

Ingredients:

- 1 cup frozen mixed LOW FODMAP berries
- 1/2 cup lactose-free yogurt
- 1/2 cup unsweetened almond milk
- 1 tbsp chia seeds
- 1/2 tsp vanilla extract
- 1/4 cup low-FODMAP granola
- 1 tbsp almonds, sliced

Directions:

- In a blender, combine the frozen mixed berries, lactose-free yogurt, almond milk, chia seeds, and vanilla extract. Blend until smooth and creamy.
- Pour the smoothie mixture into a bowl and top with low-FODMAP granola and sliced almonds.

Substitution ideas: You can replace lactose-free milk with plant-based milk such as almond or soy milk (made from isolated soy proteins). When choosing low-FODMAP berries, start with strawberries, blueberries, and raspberries.

Nutrition Information (per serving): Calories: 341, Protein: 10.7g, Fat: 15.6g, Carbohydrates: 39.4g, Fiber: 12.3g, Sugar: 18.3g

Day 16 - Lunch: Low-FODMAP Tuna Salad Lettuce Wraps

Description: A light and protein-packed lunch option, featuring tuna salad wrapped in crisp lettuce leaves.

Preparation and Cooking Time: 15 minutes

Number of Servings: 2

Ingredients:

- 1 can (5 oz) tuna in water, drained
- 1/4 cup cucumber, diced
- 1/4 cup red bell pepper, diced
- 2 tbsp plain mayonnaise
- 1 tbsp fresh parsley, chopped
- 1/3 pc lemon, juiced
- Salt and pepper, to taste
- 4 large lettuce leaves (Bibb, butter, or iceberg)

Directions:

- In a bowl, combine the drained tuna, cucumber, red bell pepper, mayonnaise, parsley, and lemon juice. Season with salt and pepper to taste and mix well.
- Spoon the tuna salad onto the lettuce leaves and fold them over to create wraps.

Nutrition Information (per serving): Calories: 214, Protein: 20.8g, Fat: 12.7g, Carbohydrates: 2.8g, Fiber: 0.6g, Sugar: 1.5g

Day 16 - Dinner: Low-FODMAP Teriyaki Chicken with Rice and Vegetables

Description: A savory and satisfying meal of teriyaki-glazed chicken served over rice with a side of colorful vegetables.

Preparation and Cooking Time: 30 minutes

Number of Servings: 4

Ingredients:

For the sauce:

- 1/2 cup low-sodium soy sauce (gluten-free)
- 1/4 cup rice vinegar
- 1/4 cup maple syrup
- 1/4 cup water
- 1 tbsp grated fresh ginger
- 1 tbsp cornstarch

- 1 lb or 4 boneless, skinless chicken breasts
- Salt and pepper to taste
- 2 tbsp olive oil
- 4 cups brown rice
- 4 cups steamed mixed vegetables (carrots, green beans, and bell peppers)
- 1/4 cup green onions (green tops only), chopped

Directions:

- In a small saucepan, whisk together the soy sauce, rice vinegar, maple syrup, water, ginger, garlic, and cornstarch. Bring the mixture to a simmer over medium heat, whisking constantly until the sauce thickens about 2-3 minutes. Remove from heat and set aside.
- Season the chicken breasts with salt and pepper. Heat olive oil in a large skillet over medium-high heat. Cook the chicken for 5-6 minutes per side, or until cooked through and the internal temperature reaches 165°F (75°C).
- Once the chicken is cooked, brush each breast with the teriyaki sauce, reserving some sauce for drizzling over the finished dish.
- To serve, divide the cooked rice and steamed vegetables between four plates. Place a teriyaki-glazed chicken breast on each plate and drizzle with additional teriyaki sauce. Garnish with chopped green onion tops.

Nutrition Information (per serving): Calories: 496, Protein: 34.7g, Fat: 10.2g, Carbohydrates: 66.1g, Fiber: 10.7g, Sugar: 13.9g

Day 17

Day 17 - Breakfast: Low-FODMAP Chia Seed Pudding with Mixed Berries

Description: A creamy and delicious chia seed pudding, topped with a variety of low-FODMAP mixed berries.

Preparation and Cooking Time: 10 minutes (plus overnight refrigeration)

Number of Servings: 2

Ingredients:
- 1/4 cup chia seeds
- 1 cup unsweetened almond milk
- 1/2 cup lactose-free yogurt
- 1 tbsp maple syrup
- 1/2 tsp vanilla extract
- 1 cup mixed berries

Directions:
- In a bowl or jar, combine chia seeds, almond milk, lactose-free yogurt, maple syrup, and vanilla extract. Stir well to combine.
- Cover and refrigerate overnight, or for at least 4 hours, until the chia seeds have absorbed the liquid and created a pudding-like consistency.

- When ready to serve, divide the chia seed pudding between two bowls and top with mixed berries.

Substitution ideas: You can replace lactose-free yogurt with plant-based yogurts such as almond or soy yogurt (made from isolated soy proteins). When choosing low-FODMAP berries, start with strawberries, blueberries, and raspberries.

Nutrition Information (per serving): Calories: 264, Protein: 7.8g, Fat: 12.7g, Carbohydrates: 31.1g, Fiber: 12.7g, Sugar: 13.9g

Day 17 - Lunch: Low-FODMAP Caprese Salad with Grilled Chicken

Description: A classic Italian Caprese salad with the addition of grilled chicken for a protein-packed and satisfying lunch.

Preparation and Cooking Time: 25 minutes

Number of Servings: 2

Ingredients:
- ½ lb or 2 boneless, skinless chicken breasts
- 1 tbsp olive oil
- Salt and pepper, to taste
- 4 cups mixed greens
- 1 cup cherry tomatoes, halved
- 4 oz fresh mozzarella cheese, sliced
- 1/4 cup fresh basil leaves
- 2 tbsp balsamic glaze

Directions:

- Preheat the grill or grill pan to medium-high heat. Brush chicken breasts with olive oil and season with salt and pepper.
- Grill the chicken for 6-8 minutes per side, or until cooked through and the internal temperature reaches 165°F (75°C). Remove from grill and let rest for a few minutes before slicing.
- On two plates, layer the mixed greens, cherry tomatoes, mozzarella cheese, and basil leaves. Top with sliced grilled chicken and drizzle with balsamic glaze.

Note: In choosing balsamic glaze, check the ingredient's nutrition label list. Watch out for onion or garlic or honey since these ingredients have high FODMAP content.

Nutrition Information (per serving): Calories: 427, Protein: 44.9g, Fat: 18.7g, Carbohydrates: 21.6g, Fiber: 3.1g, Sugar: 8.4g

Day 17- Dinner: Low-FODMAP Shrimp and Vegetable Stir-Fry

Description: A quick and easy stir-fry packed with succulent shrimp and a colorful array of vegetables, all cooked in a savory low-FODMAP sauce.

Preparation and Cooking Time: 30 minutes

Number of Servings: 4

Ingredients:
- 1 lb medium shrimp, peeled and deveined
- 2 tbsp olive oil, divided
- 1 cup red bell pepper, chopped
- 1 cup zucchini, chopped

- ½ cup green onions (green tops only), chopped
- 1/2 cup carrots, chopped
- 1/4 cup low-sodium soy sauce (gluten-free)
- 2 tbsp rice vinegar
- 1 tbsp maple syrup
- 1 tbsp cornstarch
- 1/4 tsp crushed red pepper flakes (optional)
- 2 cups cooked brown rice

Directions:

- In a large skillet or wok, heat 1 tablespoon of olive oil over medium-high heat. Add the shrimp and cook for 2-3 minutes per side, or until cooked through and pink. Remove shrimp from the skillet and set aside.
- In the same skillet, heat the remaining tablespoon of olive oil. Add the red bell pepper, zucchini, green onion tops, and carrots, and cook for 5-7 minutes, or until the vegetables are tender-crisp.
- In a small bowl, whisk together the low-sodium soy sauce, rice vinegar, maple syrup, cornstarch, and crushed red pepper flakes (if using) to create the stir-fry sauce.
- Add the cooked shrimp back to the skillet with the vegetables, and pour the sauce over the top. Stir to combine and cook for an additional 2-3 minutes, until the sauce has thickened and everything is heated through.
- Serve the shrimp and vegetable stir-fry over cooked rice.

Nutrition Information (per serving): Calories: 330, Protein: 29.6g, Fat: 9.7g, Carbohydrates: 29.7g, Fiber: 1.9g, Sugar: 6.9g

Day 18

Day 18- Breakfast: Low-FODMAP Berry Smoothie Bowl

Description: A refreshing and filling berry smoothie bowl that's perfect for a quick and easy breakfast.

Preparation and Cooking Time: 10 minutes

Number of Servings: 1

Ingredients:
- 1 cup lactose-free yogurt
- 1/2 cup frozen mixed berries
- 1/2 "just ripe" banana
- 1 tbsp chia seeds
- 1/4 cup low-FODMAP granola
- Additional berries for topping (optional)

Directions:
- In a blender, combine the lactose-free yogurt, frozen mixed berries, and half a banana. Blend until smooth and creamy.
- Pour the smoothie into a bowl and top with chia seeds, low-FODMAP granola, and additional berries if desired.
- Enjoy immediately.

Substitution ideas: You can replace lactose-free yogurt with plant-based yogurts such as almond or soy yogurt (made from isolated soy proteins). When choosing low-FODMAP berries, start with strawberries, blueberries, and raspberries.

Nutrition Information (per serving): Calories: 340, Protein: 12.9g, Fat: 12.8g, Carbohydrates: 47.5g, Fiber: 9.9g, Sugar: 24.1g

Day 18- Lunch: Quinoa and Roasted Vegetable Salad

Description: A healthy and satisfying salad packed with protein-rich quinoa and roasted vegetables.

Preparation and Cooking Time: 40 minutes

Number of Servings: 4

Ingredients:

- 1 cup quinoa, uncooked
- 2 cups water
- 1 medium zucchini, sliced
- 1 medium red bell pepper, chopped
- 1 cup cherry tomatoes, halved
- 2 tbsp olive oil, divided
- Salt and pepper, to taste
- 2 cups baby spinach
- 1/4 cup fresh parsley, chopped
- 1/4 cup green onions (green tops only), chopped
- 2/3 pc lemon, juiced
- 1/4 cup feta cheese, crumbled

Directions:

- Preheat oven to 400°F (200°C). Cook quinoa according to package instructions with 2 cups of water. Set aside.
- On a large baking sheet, toss the zucchini, red bell pepper, and cherry tomatoes with 1 tablespoon of olive oil. Season with salt and pepper. Roast for 25-30 minutes, or until the vegetables are tender and lightly browned.

- In a large bowl, combine the cooked quinoa, roasted vegetables, baby spinach, parsley, and green onion tops. Drizzle with the remaining tablespoon of olive oil and lemon juice. Toss to combine.
- Serve the salad warm or at room temperature, topped with crumbled feta cheese if desired.

Nutrition Information (per serving): Calories: 275, Protein: 9.3g, Fat: 12g, Carbohydrates: 34.7g, Fiber: 5.1g, Sugar: 4.3g

Day 18-Dinner: Low-FODMAP Chicken Alfredo

Description: A creamy and delicious low-FODMAP version of the classic Chicken Alfredo.

Preparation and Cooking Time: 30 minutes

Number of Servings: 4

Ingredients:

- 8 oz gluten-free fettuccine
- 2 tbsp olive oil, divided
- 1 lb boneless, skinless chicken breasts, thinly sliced
- Salt and pepper, to taste
- 2 cups lactose-free milk
- 2 tbsp cornstarch
- 1/2 cup Parmesan cheese, grated
- 1/4 cup fresh parsley, chopped
- 1/4 cup green onions (green tops only), chopped

Directions:

- Cook the gluten-free fettuccine according to package instructions. Drain and set aside.

- In a large skillet, heat 1 tablespoon of olive oil over medium heat. Season the chicken with salt and pepper, and cook for 5-6 minutes per side or until cooked through. Remove from the skillet and set aside.
- In the same skillet, heat the remaining 1 tablespoon of olive oil. Add the lactose-free milk and bring to a simmer. Whisk in the cornstarch, stirring constantly until the sauce thickens.
- Stir in the grated Parmesan cheese and continue to cook until the cheese is melted and the sauce is smooth.
- Add the cooked fettuccine, chicken, parsley, and green onion tops to the skillet. Toss everything together until well combined and heated through.
- Serve the Chicken Alfredo immediately, garnished with additional parsley and Parmesan cheese if desired.

Substitution ideas: You can replace lactose-free milk with plant-based milk such as almond or soy milk (made from isolated soy proteins).

Nutrition Information (per serving): Calories: 495, Protein: 40.7g, Fat: 17.6g, Carbohydrates: 47.1g, Fiber: 2.6g, Sugar: 6.2g

Day 19

Day 19- Breakfast: Low-FODMAP Overnight Oats

Description: A simple and delicious make-ahead breakfast that's perfect for busy mornings.

Preparation and Cooking Time: 5 minutes (plus overnight refrigeration)

Number of Servings: 1

Ingredients:

- 1/2 cup rolled oats
- 1/2 cup lactose-free yogurt
- 1/2 cup lactose-free milk
- 1 tbsp chia seeds
- 1 tbsp pure maple syrup
- 1/2 cup strawberries, diced
- 1/4 cup blueberries

Directions:

- In a mason jar or airtight container, combine the rolled oats, lactose-free yogurt, lactose-free milk, chia seeds, and maple syrup. Stir well to combine.
- Top with the diced strawberries and blueberries.
- Seal the container with a lid and refrigerate overnight (or for at least 4 hours).
- In the morning, give the oats a good stir and enjoy it cold.

Substitution ideas: You can replace lactose-free milk/yogurt with plant-based milk/yogurt such as almond or soy milk/yogurt (made from isolated soy proteins).

Nutrition Information (per serving): Calories: 391, Protein: 14.4g, Fat: 9.5g, Carbohydrates: 64.1g, Fiber: 6.5g, Sugar: 31.2g

Day 19- Lunch: Low-FODMAP Veggie Wrap

Description: A light and refreshing veggie wrap that's perfect for a quick and healthy lunch.

Preparation and Cooking Time: 15 minutes

Number of Servings: 2

Ingredients:
- 2 large gluten-free tortillas
- 1/2 cup lactose-free cream cheese
- 1 cup baby spinach leaves
- 1 small cucumber, thinly sliced
- 1 medium carrot, grated
- 1/2 cup red bell pepper, thinly sliced
- 1/4 cup green onions (green tops only), chopped

Directions:
- Lay the gluten-free tortillas on a flat surface. Spread each tortilla with 1/4 cup of lactose-free cream cheese.
- Divide the baby spinach, cucumber slices, grated carrot, red bell pepper slices, and green onion tops evenly between the two tortillas.
- Roll up the tortillas tightly, tucking in the ends as you go.
- Slice each wrap in half and serve immediately.

Substitution ideas: You can use corn tortillas as your gluten-free flour.

Nutrition Information (per serving): Calories: 384, Protein: 8.6g, Fat: 24.6g, Carbohydrates: 37.7g, Fiber: 4.6g, Sugar: 7g

Day 19- Dinner: Low-FODMAP Grilled Lemon-Herb Chicken

Description: A flavorful and tender grilled chicken dish that's perfect for a healthy and satisfying dinner.

Preparation and Cooking Time: 30 minutes (plus at least 30 mins to 4 hours of marinating time)

Number of Servings: 4

Ingredients:

- 1/4 cup olive oil
- 1 1/3 pc lemon, juiced
- 2 tbsp chopped fresh parsley
- 1 tbsp chopped fresh basil
- 1 tbsp chopped fresh oregano
- 1/2 tsp salt
- 1/4 tsp black pepper
- 4 boneless, skinless chicken breasts

Directions:

- In a small bowl, whisk together the olive oil, lemon juice, parsley, basil, oregano, salt, and pepper.
- Place the chicken breasts in a shallow dish or resealable plastic bag. Pour the marinade over the chicken, making sure each piece is well-coated. Cover or seal and refrigerate for at least 30 minutes or up to 4 hours.
- Preheat a grill or grill pan over medium-high heat. Remove the chicken from the marinade, discarding any excess marinade.
- Grill the chicken for 5-6 minutes per side or until cooked through and the internal temperature reaches 165°F (74°C).
- Let the chicken rest for a few minutes before serving. Enjoy with your favorite low-FODMAP side dishes.

Nutrition Information (per serving): Calories: 236, Protein: 26.3g, Fat: 14.4g, Carbohydrates: 1.3g, Fiber: 0.6g, Sugar: 0.4g

Day 20

Day 20- Breakfast: Low-FODMAP Spinach and Feta Frittata

Description: A savory and satisfying frittata that's perfect for a quick and easy breakfast or brunch.

Preparation and Cooking Time: 30 minutes

Number of Servings: 4

Ingredients:

- 8 large eggs
- 1/4 cup lactose-free milk
- Salt and pepper, to taste
- 2 tbsp olive oil
- 1/4 cup green onions (green tops only), chopped
- 1 cup baby spinach leaves
- 1/2 cup feta cheese, crumbled

Directions:

- In a large bowl, whisk together the eggs, lactose-free milk, salt, and pepper. Set aside.
- Preheat the oven to 350°F (180°C). In an oven-safe skillet, heat the olive oil over medium heat. Add the green onion tops and cook for 2-3 minutes or until softened.
- Add the spinach to the skillet and cook for 1-2 minutes or until wilted.
- Pour the egg mixture over the spinach and green onions, stirring gently to distribute the ingredients evenly. Cook for 3-4 minutes or until the edges of the frittata are set.

- Sprinkle the crumbled feta cheese evenly over the top of the frittata.
- Transfer the skillet to the oven and bake for 12-15 minutes or until the frittata is cooked through and the cheese is slightly browned.
- Remove from the oven and let the frittata rest for a few minutes before cutting into wedges and serving.

Substitution ideas: You can replace lactose-free milk with plant-based milk such as almond or soy milk (made from isolated soy proteins).

Nutrition Information (per serving): Calories: 264, Protein: 16.1g, Fat: 21.3g, Carbohydrates: 3.1g, Fiber: 0.3g, Sugar: 2.5g

Day 20- Lunch: Low-FODMAP Tuna Salad Lettuce Wraps

Description: A light and refreshing lunch option that's packed with protein and flavor.

Preparation and Cooking Time: 15 minutes

Number of Servings: 2

Ingredients:
- 1 can (5 oz) canned tuna in water, drained
- 1/4 cup lactose-free plain mayonnaise
- 1/4 cup red bell pepper, diced
- 1/4 cup green onions (green tops only), chopped
- 1/4 cup fresh parsley, chopped
- Salt and pepper, to taste
- 4 large lettuce leaves (such as romaine or butter lettuce)

Directions:

- In a medium bowl, combine the drained tuna, lactose-free mayonnaise, diced red bell pepper, green onion tops, and parsley. Stir until well combined. Season with salt and pepper to taste.
- Lay the lettuce leaves on a flat surface. Divide the tuna salad evenly among the leaves.
- Roll up the lettuce leaves, tucking in the ends as you go. Secure with a toothpick if necessary.
- Serve the tuna salad lettuce wraps immediately.

Nutrition Information (per serving): Calories: 306, Protein: 21.1g, Fat: 22.7g, Carbohydrates: 3.5g, Fiber: 1g, Sugar: 1.4g

Day 20- Dinner: Low-FODMAP Shrimp Stir-Fry

Description: A flavorful and colorful stir-fry dish that's quick to prepare and perfect for a weeknight dinner.

Preparation and Cooking Time: 30 minutes

Number of Servings: 4

Ingredients:

- 1 lb medium shrimp, peeled and deveined
- Salt and pepper, to taste
- 2 tbsp olive oil, divided
- 1 medium zucchini, sliced
- 1 medium red bell pepper, sliced
- 1/2 cup green onion tops (green part only), chopped
- 1/4 cup low-sodium soy sauce (gluten-free)
- 1 tbsp fresh ginger, grated
- 2 cups cooked brown rice

Directions:

- Season the shrimp with salt and pepper.
- In a large skillet or wok, heat 1 tablespoon of olive oil over medium-high heat. Add the shrimp and cook for 2-3 minutes per side or until pink and cooked through. Remove the shrimp from the skillet and set aside.
- In the same skillet, heat the remaining 1 tablespoon of olive oil. Add the zucchini, red bell pepper, and green onion tops, and stir-fry for 5-6 minutes or until the vegetables are tender-crisp.
- Return the shrimp to the skillet. Add the soy sauce and grated ginger, and stir to combine. Cook for an additional 2-3 minutes or until everything is heated through and well combined.
- Serve the shrimp stir-fry over cooked white or brown rice.

Nutrition Information (per serving): Calories: 359, Protein: 30.5g, Fat: 10.1g, Carbohydrates: 41.8g, Fiber: 3.5g, Sugar: 3.7g

Day 21

Day 21- Breakfast: Low-FODMAP Peanut Butter Banana Smoothie

Description: A creamy, filling smoothie with a delicious combination of peanut butter and banana.

Preparation and Cooking Time: 5 minutes

Number of Servings: 2

Ingredients:

- 2 "just ripe" bananas
- 1 cup lactose-free milk or unsweetened almond milk
- 1/4 cup natural plain peanut butter
- 1/4 tsp cinnamon
- 1 tbsp chia seeds
- 1 cup ice

Directions:

- In a blender, combine the bananas, lactose-free milk, peanut butter, cinnamon, chia seeds, and ice.
- Blend until smooth and creamy.
- Pour the smoothie into two glasses and serve immediately.

Nutrition Information (per serving): Calories: 395, Protein: 14.5g, Fat: 21.3g, Carbohydrates: 43g, Fiber: 7.6g, Sugar: 23.5g

Day 21 Lunch: Low-FODMAP Spinach and Feta Stuffed Chicken Breast

Description: A flavorful and satisfying lunch that combines tender chicken breast with delicious spinach and feta stuffing.

Preparation and Cooking Time: 35 minutes

Number of Servings: 4

Ingredients:

- 1 lb or 4 boneless, skinless chicken breasts
- 2 cups fresh spinach, chopped
- 1/2 cup feta cheese, crumbled
- 1/4 cup lactose-free cream cheese
- 1/4 tsp garlic-infused olive oil

- Salt and pepper, to taste

Directions:

- Preheat the oven to 375°F (190°C).
- Using a sharp knife, cut a pocket into each chicken breast, being careful not to cut all the way through.
- In a medium bowl, combine the spinach, feta cheese, cream cheese, and garlic-infused olive oil. Season with salt and pepper to taste.
- Stuff each chicken breast pocket with the spinach and feta mixture, dividing it evenly.
- Place the stuffed chicken breasts in a baking dish and bake for 20-25 minutes or until the chicken is cooked through and no longer pink in the center.
- Remove from the oven and serve immediately.

Nutrition Information (per serving): Calories: 226, Protein: 30.2g, Fat: 10.9g, Carbohydrates: 1.7g, Fiber: 0.3g, Sugar: 0.9g

Day 21 Dinner: Low-FODMAP Sesame Ginger Salmon

Description: A delicious, Asian-inspired salmon dish with a flavorful sesame ginger glaze.

Preparation and Cooking Time: 20 minutes

Number of Servings: 4

Ingredients:

- 4 (6 oz each) salmon fillets
- 3 tbsp tamari or gluten-free soy sauce
- 1 tbsp fresh grated ginger

- 1 tbsp sesame oil
- 1 tbsp rice vinegar
- 1 tbsp maple syrup
- 2 tbsp sesame seeds
- Green onions (green tops only), sliced for garnish

Directions:

- Preheat the oven to 425°F (220°C).
- Place the salmon fillets on a lined baking sheet.
- In a small bowl, whisk together the tamari, ginger, sesame oil, rice vinegar, and maple syrup.
- Brush the salmon fillets with the sesame ginger sauce, reserving some for serving.
- Sprinkle the salmon fillets with sesame seeds.
- Bake the salmon in the preheated oven for 12-15 minutes or until the salmon flakes easily with a fork.
- Remove from the oven and garnish with green onion tops.
- Serve the salmon with reserved sesame ginger sauce on the side.

Nutrition Information (per serving): Calories: 356, Protein: 43.3g, Fat: 17.8g, Carbohydrates: 6.1g, Fiber: 0.8g, Sugar: 3.3g

Day 22

Day 22-Breakfast: Low-FODMAP Veggie Omelette

Description: A delicious and protein-packed omelette filled with sautéed vegetables.

Preparation and Cooking Time: 20 minutes

Number of Servings: 2

Ingredients:

- 4 large eggs
- 1/4 cup lactose-free milk
- Salt and pepper, to taste
- 1 tbsp olive oil
- 1/2 cup red bell pepper, diced
- 1/2 cup green onions (green tops only), chopped
- 1/2 cup spinach, chopped
- 1/4 cup feta cheese, crumbled

Directions:

- In a medium bowl, whisk together the eggs, lactose-free milk, salt, and pepper.
- Heat the olive oil in a non-stick skillet over medium heat. Add the red bell pepper and green onion tops, and sauté for 3-4 minutes, or until softened.
- Add the chopped spinach to the skillet and cook for an additional 1-2 minutes, or until the spinach is wilted.
- Pour the egg mixture over the vegetables in the skillet, ensuring they are evenly distributed.
- Sprinkle the crumbled feta cheese over the top of the omelette.
- Cook the omelette for 4-5 minutes, or until the edges are set and the center is still slightly soft.
- Carefully fold the omelette in half and continue to cook for another 1-2 minutes, or until the center is fully set.
- Slide the omelette onto a plate and serve immediately.

Substitution ideas: You can replace lactose-free milk with plant-based milk such as almond or soy milk (made from isolated soy proteins).

Nutrition Information (per serving): Calories: 288, Protein: 17.2g, Fat: 21.7g, Carbohydrates: 7.6g, Fiber: 1.2g, Sugar: 5.2g

Day 22- Lunch: Low-FODMAP Greek Salad with Grilled Chicken

Description: A fresh and flavorful Greek salad topped with grilled chicken for a satisfying and healthy lunch.

Preparation and Cooking Time: 20 minutes

Number of Servings: 4

Ingredients:

- 1 lb or 4 boneless, skinless chicken breasts
- Salt and pepper, to taste
- 4 cups Romaine lettuce, chopped
- 1 cup cherry tomatoes, halved
- 1 cup cucumber, diced
- 1/2 cup Kalamata olives, pitted
- 1/2 cup feta cheese, crumbled

For the dressing:

- 1/4 cup olive oil
- 2 tbsp red wine vinegar
- 1/3 pc lemon, juiced
- 1/2 tsp dried oregano
- Salt and pepper, to taste

Directions:

- Preheat a grill or grill pan to medium-high heat. Season the chicken breasts with salt and pepper.
- Grill the chicken for 5-6 minutes per side, or until cooked through and no longer pink in the center. Remove from the grill and let rest for a few minutes before slicing.
- In a large bowl, combine the Romaine lettuce, cherry tomatoes, cucumber, Kalamata olives, and feta cheese. Toss to mix.

- To make the dressing, whisk together the olive oil, red wine vinegar, lemon juice, dried oregano, salt, and pepper in a small bowl.
- Drizzle the dressing over the salad and toss to coat.
- Divide the salad among four plates and top each with a sliced grilled chicken breast.
- Serve immediately.

Nutrition Information (per serving): Calories: 319, Protein: 29.7g, Fat: 20.2g, Carbohydrates: 6.5g, Fiber: 1.7g, Sugar: 3.1g

Day 22- Dinner: Low-FODMAP Shrimp and Vegetable Stir-Fry

Description: A quick and delicious stir-fry featuring shrimp and a variety of colorful vegetables.

Preparation and Cooking Time: 25 minutes

Number of Servings: 4

Ingredients:
- 1 lb large shrimp, peeled and deveined
- 1 tbsp garlic-infused olive oil
- 1/4 cup tamari or gluten-free soy sauce
- 2 tbsp rice vinegar
- 1 tbsp maple syrup
- 1/2 tsp ground ginger
- 2 cups bell peppers (various colors), chopped
- 1 cup zucchini, chopped
- 1/2 cup green onions (green tops only), chopped
- 1/4 cup fresh cilantro, chopped
- 1 tbsp sesame seeds

Directions:

- In a large skillet, heat the garlic-infused olive oil over medium-high heat. Add the shrimp and cook for 2-3 minutes per side, or until pink and cooked through. Remove the shrimp from the skillet and set aside.
- In a small bowl, whisk together the tamari, rice vinegar, maple syrup, and ground ginger. Set aside.
- In the same skillet, add the bell peppers and zucchini. Cook for 4-5 minutes, or until the vegetables are tender-crisp.
- Add the cooked shrimp back to the skillet along with the tamari sauce mixture. Cook for an additional 1-2 minutes, stirring to coat the shrimp and vegetables in the sauce.
- Remove the skillet from the heat and stir in the green onion tops and chopped cilantro.
- Serve the shrimp and vegetable stir-fry over cooked rice or low-FODMAP noodles, if desired. Sprinkle with sesame seeds before serving.

Nutrition Information (per serving): Calories: 221, Protein: 26.6g, Fat: 6.9g, Carbohydrates: 11.5g, Fiber: 1.9g, Sugar: 7.1g

Day 23

Day 23- Breakfast: Low-FODMAP Blueberry Banana Smoothie

Description: A refreshing and fruity smoothie to start your day.

Preparation and Cooking Time: 5 minutes

Number of Servings: 1

Ingredients:

- 1/2 "just ripe" banana, sliced and frozen
- 1/2 cup frozen blueberries
- 1 cup lactose-free yogurt
- 1/2 cup unsweetened almond milk
- 1 tbsp chia seeds

Directions:

- In a blender, combine the frozen banana, blueberries, yogurt, almond milk, and chia seeds.
- Blend until smooth and creamy.
- Pour into a glass and enjoy immediately.

Substitution ideas: You can replace lactose-free yogurt with plant-based yogurts such as coconut, almond, or soy yogurt (made from isolated soy proteins).

Nutrition Information (per serving): Calories: 321, Protein: 11.9g, Fat: 13.9g, Carbohydrates: 41.5g, Fiber: 8.7g, Sugar: 25g

Day 23- Lunch: Low-FODMAP Chicken Caesar Salad Wrap

Description: A classic Caesar salad with grilled chicken, wrapped in a low-FODMAP tortilla for a delicious and portable lunch.

Preparation and Cooking Time: 15 minutes

Number of Servings: 2

Ingredients:

- 2 low-FODMAP tortillas
- ½ lb or 2 grilled chicken breasts, sliced
- 4 cups Romaine lettuce, chopped

- 1/4 cup Parmesan cheese, grated
- 1/4 cup low-FODMAP Caesar dressing

Directions:

- In a large bowl, combine the sliced grilled chicken, Romaine lettuce, Parmesan cheese, and Caesar dressing. Toss to combine.
- Divide the chicken Caesar salad mixture between the two tortillas, placing it in the center of each tortilla.
- Fold the sides of the tortilla over the salad mixture, then roll the wrap tightly.
- Cut each wrap in half and serve immediately.

Substitution ideas: You can use corn tortillas as your gluten-free flour.

Note: In choosing Caesar Dressing, check the ingredient's nutrition label list. Watch out for onion or garlic since these ingredients have high FODMAP content.

Nutrition Information (per serving): Calories: 498, Protein: 41.7g, Fat: 23.8g, Carbohydrates: 28.3g, Fiber: 0.7g, Sugar: 3.1g

Day 23- Dinner: Low-FODMAP Vegetable Frittata

Description: A colorful and protein-packed frittata filled with a variety of low-FODMAP vegetables.

Preparation and Cooking Time: 30 minutes

Number of Servings: 4

Ingredients:

- 8 large eggs
- 1/4 cup lactose-free milk

- Salt and pepper, to taste
- 2 tbsp garlic-infused olive oil
- 1 cup bell peppers, diced
- 1 cup zucchini, diced
- 1/2 cup green onions (green tops only), chopped
- 1/2 cup Parmesan cheese, grated

Directions:

- Preheat the oven to 375°F (190°C).
- In a large bowl, whisk together the eggs, milk, salt, and pepper. Set aside.
- In a large ovenproof skillet, heat the garlic-infused olive oil over medium heat. Add the bell peppers and zucchini, and cook for 5 minutes, or until the vegetables are tender.
- Stir in the green onion tops, then pour the egg mixture over the vegetables. Cook for 3-4 minutes, or until the edges of the frittata are set.
- Sprinkle the Parmesan cheese over the top of the frittata, then transfer the skillet to the preheated oven. Bake for 10-12 minutes, or until the frittata is set in the center and the cheese is melted and bubbly.
- Remove the skillet from the oven and let the frittata cool for a few minutes before slicing and serving.

Substitution ideas: You can replace lactose-free milk with plant-based milk such as almond or soy milk (made from isolated soy proteins).

Nutrition Information (per serving): Calories: 319, Protein: 23g, Fat: 23.4g, Carbohydrates: 6.7g, Fiber: 1.1g, Sugar: 3.8g

Day 24

Day 24- Breakfast: Low-FODMAP Overnight Oats with Strawberries and Almonds

Description: Creamy and delicious overnight oats with a hint of sweetness from the strawberries and a satisfying crunch from the almonds.

Preparation and Cooking Time: 5 minutes (plus overnight refrigeration)

Number of Servings: 1

Ingredients:

- 1/2 cup rolled oats
- 3/4 cup unsweetened almond milk
- 1/2 cup strawberries, chopped
- 2 tbsp almonds, chopped
- 1 tbsp maple syrup

Directions:

- In a mason jar or airtight container, combine the rolled oats, almond milk, chopped strawberries, chopped almonds, and maple syrup.
- Stir well to combine, then cover and refrigerate overnight.
- In the morning, give the oats a good stir and enjoy.

Nutrition Information (per serving): Calories: 329, Protein: 9.1g, Fat: 11.5g, Carbohydrates: 50.7g, Fiber: 7.8g, Sugar: 16.3g

Day 24- Lunch: Low-FODMAP Greek Salad with Quinoa

Description: A light and refreshing Greek salad with the added benefits of protein-rich quinoa.

Preparation and Cooking Time: 25 minutes

Number of Servings: 4

Ingredients:

- 1 cup quinoa, uncooked, rinsed, and drained
- 2 cups water
- 4 cups Romaine lettuce, chopped
- 1 cup cucumber, diced
- 1 cup red bell pepper, diced
- 1/2 cup Kalamata olives, pitted & halved
- 1/2 cup feta cheese, crumbled
- 1/4 cup green onions (green tops only), chopped
- 1/4 cup low-FODMAP Greek dressing

Directions:

- In a medium saucepan, combine the quinoa and water. Bring to a boil, then reduce the heat to low, cover, and simmer for 15 minutes, or until the quinoa is tender and the water has been absorbed.
- Remove the saucepan from the heat and let the quinoa cool for a few minutes.
- In a large bowl, combine the Romaine lettuce, cucumber, red bell pepper, olives, feta cheese, and green onion tops.
- Add the cooled quinoa and Greek dressing to the salad, tossing to combine.
- Serve immediately or chill for later use.

Note: In choosing Greek Dressing, check the ingredient's nutrition label list. Watch out for onion or garlic since these ingredients have high FODMAP content.

Nutrition Information (per serving): Calories: 308, Protein: 9.8g, Fat: 14.6g, Carbohydrates: 35.9g, Fiber: 4.6g, Sugar: 4.4g

Day 24-Dinner: Low-FODMAP Lemon Herb Chicken with Roasted Carrots

Description: Flavorful lemon herb chicken served with tender, roasted carrots.

Preparation and Cooking Time: 45 minutes

Number of Servings: 4

Ingredients:

- 1 lb or 4 boneless, skinless chicken breasts
- 1/4 cup garlic-infused olive oil
- 1 pc lemon, juiced
- 2 tsp dried oregano
- 2 tsp dried basil
- Salt and pepper, to taste
- 1 lb carrots, peeled and cut into 1-inch pieces

Directions:

- Preheat the oven to 400°F (200°C).
- In a small bowl, whisk together the garlic-infused olive oil, lemon juice, oregano, basil, salt, and pepper.
- Place the chicken breasts in a baking dish and pour the lemon herb mixture over the top, making sure each chicken breast is well coated.

- In a separate baking dish, toss the carrots with 1 tablespoon of the remaining lemon-herb mixture.
- Place both baking dishes in the preheated oven. Bake the chicken for 25-30 minutes, or until the internal temperature reaches 165°F (74°C).
- Bake the carrots for 35-40 minutes, or until tender and lightly caramelized, stirring occasionally to ensure even cooking.
- Remove both dishes from the oven and let the chicken rest for a few minutes before serving alongside the roasted carrots.

Nutrition Information (per serving): Calories: 280, Protein: 27.1g, Fat: 14.3g, Carbohydrates: 11.9g, Fiber: 3.2g, Sugar: 5.9g

Day 25

Day 25- Breakfast: Low-FODMAP Chia Pudding with Raspberry Compote

Description: A creamy chia pudding topped with a delicious homemade raspberry compote.

Preparation and Cooking Time: 10 minutes (plus overnight refrigeration)

Number of Servings: 2

Ingredients:
- 1/4 cup chia seeds
- 1 cup unsweetened almond milk
- 1 tbsp maple syrup
- 1 tsp vanilla extract

- 1 cup fresh or frozen raspberries
- 2 tbsp water
- 2 tbsp granulated sugar

Directions:

- In a medium bowl, whisk together the chia seeds, almond milk, maple syrup, and vanilla extract. Cover and refrigerate overnight.
- In a small saucepan, combine the raspberries, water, and sugar. Cook over medium heat, stirring occasionally, until the raspberries have broken down and the mixture has thickened about 5 minutes. Let the compote cool.
- In the morning, give the chia pudding a good stir, then divide it between two serving bowls or glasses. Top each with half of the raspberry compote and serve.

Nutrition Information (per serving): Calories: 265, Protein: 6.2g, Fat: 10.5g, Carbohydrates: 38.9g, Fiber: 12.2g, Sugar: 21.7g

Day 25- Lunch: Low-FODMAP Caprese Salad with Grilled Chicken

Description: A classic Caprese salad with juicy grilled chicken for added protein.

Preparation and Cooking Time: 20 minutes

Number of Servings: 4

Ingredients:

- 1 lb or 4 grilled chicken breasts, sliced
- 4 cups fresh basil leaves
- 4 large tomatoes, sliced

- 8 oz fresh mozzarella, sliced
- 1/4 cup balsamic glaze
- 1/4 cup garlic-infused olive oil
- Salt and pepper, to taste

Directions:

- Arrange the sliced grilled chicken, basil leaves, tomato slices, and mozzarella slices on a large serving platter.
- Drizzle the balsamic glaze and garlic-infused olive oil over the salad. Season with salt and pepper to taste.
- Serve immediately.

Note: In choosing balsamic glaze, check the ingredient's nutrition label list. Watch out for honey, onion, or garlic since these ingredients have high FODMAP content.

Nutrition Information (per serving): Calories: 504, Protein: 47.6g, Fat: 30.7g, Carbohydrates: 13.7g, Fiber: 4.6g, Sugar: 7.9g

Day 25- Dinner: Low-FODMAP Shrimp and Vegetable Stir-Fry

Description: A quick and easy shrimp stir-fry with a medley of low-FODMAP vegetables.

Preparation and Cooking Time: 25 minutes

Number of Servings: 4

Ingredients:

- 1 lb shrimp, peeled and deveined
- 2 tbsp garlic-infused olive oil, divided
- 1 cup red bell pepper, diced

- 1 cup zucchini, diced
- 1 cup cherry tomatoes, halved
- 1/4 cup green onions (green tops only), chopped
- 1/4 cup low-sodium soy sauce (gluten-free)
- 1 tbsp rice vinegar
- 1 tbsp maple syrup
- 1 tsp cornstarch
- Salt and pepper, to taste
- 2 cups cooked jasmine/white rice, for serving

Directions:

- In a large skillet or wok, heat 1 tablespoon of garlic-infused olive oil over medium-high heat. Add the shrimp and cook for 2-3 minutes per side, or until they are pink and opaque. Remove the shrimp from the skillet and set aside.
- In the same skillet, heat the remaining 1 tablespoon of garlic-infused olive oil. Add the red bell pepper and zucchini, cooking for 5-7 minutes, or until the vegetables are tender-crisp.
- Add the cherry tomatoes and green onion tops to the skillet, and cook for an additional 2 minutes.
- In a small bowl, whisk together the soy sauce, rice vinegar, maple syrup, and cornstarch. Pour the sauce into the skillet with the vegetables, stirring to coat. Cook for 1-2 minutes, or until the sauce has thickened slightly.
- Return the cooked shrimp to the skillet, tossing to combine and heat through. Season with salt and pepper to taste.
- Serve the shrimp and vegetable stir-fry over cooked jasmine rice.

Nutrition Information (per serving): Calories: 402, Protein: 30.5g, Fat: 13g, Carbohydrates: 41.5g, Fiber: 2.1g, Sugar: 7.3g

Day 26

Day 26- Breakfast: Low-FODMAP Almond Butter and Banana Toast

Description: A simple yet satisfying breakfast toast with creamy almond butter and sliced banana.

Preparation and Cooking Time: 5 minutes

Number of Servings: 1

Ingredients:

- 2 slices gluten-free bread, toasted
- 2 tbsp almond butter
- 1 small "just ripe" banana, sliced
- 1 tbsp chia seeds

Directions:

- Spread 1 tablespoon of almond butter on each slice of toasted low-FODMAP bread.
- Arrange the banana slices evenly over the almond butter, then sprinkle with chia seeds.
- Enjoy immediately.

Nutrition Information (per serving): Calories: 575, Protein: 13.2g, Fat: 26.2g, Carbohydrates: 78g, Fiber: 11.7g, Sugar: 16.8g

Day 26- Lunch: Low-FODMAP Spinach and Feta Stuffed Chicken Breast

Description: Tender chicken breasts stuffed with delicious spinach and feta filling.

Preparation and Cooking Time: 45 minutes

Number of Servings: 4

Ingredients:
- 1 lb or 4 boneless, skinless chicken breasts
- 1 tbsp garlic-infused olive oil
- 4 cups fresh spinach
- 1/2 cup feta cheese, crumbled
- Salt and pepper, to taste
- Toothpicks, for securing the chicken

Directions:
- Preheat the oven to 375°F (190°C).
- Using a sharp knife, create a pocket in each chicken breast by making a horizontal cut along the thickest part, being careful not to cut all the way through.
- In a large skillet, heat the garlic-infused olive oil over medium heat. Add the spinach and cook for 2-3 minutes, or until wilted. Remove the skillet from the heat and stir in the crumbled feta cheese.
- Stuff each chicken breast with the spinach and feta mixture, then secure the opening with toothpicks.
- Season the stuffed chicken breasts with salt and pepper, then place them in a baking dish.
- Bake for 25-30 minutes, or until the chicken is cooked through and the internal temperature reaches 165°F (74°C).
- Remove the toothpicks before serving.

Nutrition Information (per serving): Calories: 206, Protein: 29.5g, Fat: 9.1g, Carbohydrates: 1.9g, Fiber: 0.7g, Sugar: 0.9g

Day 26- Dinner: Low-FODMAP Vegetable Curry with Basmati Rice

Description: A fragrant and flavorful vegetable curry served over a bed of fluffy Basmati rice.

Preparation and Cooking Time: 40 minutes

Number of Servings: 4

Ingredients:

- 2 tbsp garlic-infused olive oil
- 1 tbsp grated fresh ginger
- 2 tsp ground turmeric
- 1 tsp ground cumin
- 1 tsp ground coriander
- 1/2 tsp ground cinnamon
- 1/2 tsp ground cardamom
- 1/4 tsp cayenne pepper (optional)
- 1 cup red bell pepper, diced
- 1 cup zucchini, diced
- 1 cup eggplant, diced
- 1 (14 oz) can of diced tomatoes
- 1 (14 oz) can coconut milk
- Salt and pepper, to taste
- 1/4 cup fresh cilantro, chopped
- 2 cups cooked Basmati rice, for serving

Directions:

- In a large pot, heat the garlic-infused olive oil over medium heat. Add the ginger, turmeric, cumin, coriander, cinnamon, cardamom, and cayenne pepper (if using), cooking for 1-2 minutes, or until fragrant.
- Add the red bell pepper, zucchini, and eggplant to the pot, stirring to coat the vegetables with the spices.
- Stir in the diced tomatoes and coconut milk, then bring the mixture to a simmer. Reduce the heat to low and cook, covered, for 20-25 minutes, or until the vegetables are tender.
- Season the vegetable curry with salt and pepper to taste, then stir in the chopped fresh cilantro.
- Serve the vegetable curry over cooked Basmati rice.

Nutrition Information (per serving): Calories: 459, Protein: 6.5g, Fat: 31.6g, Carbohydrates: 42.8g, Fiber: 5.8g, Sugar: 8.7g

Day 27

Day 27- Breakfast: Low-FODMAP Yogurt Parfait with Berries and Granola

Description: A delicious and nutritious yogurt parfait layered with fresh berries and crunchy granola.

Preparation and Cooking Time: 5 minutes

Number of Servings: 1

Ingredients:

- 1 cup lactose-free yogurt

- 1/2 cup mixed berries
- 1/4 cup low-FODMAP granola
- 1 tbsp maple syrup

Directions:
- In a glass or jar, layer the yogurt, mixed berries, and granola.
- Drizzle the maple syrup over the top and enjoy.

Substitution ideas: You can replace lactose-free yogurt with plant-based yogurts such as coconut, almond, or soy milk (made from isolated soy proteins). When choosing low-FODMAP berries, start with strawberries, blueberries, and raspberries.

Nutrition Information (per serving): Calories: 285, Protein: 10.4g, Fat: 8.9g, Carbohydrates: 42g, Fiber: 3.5g, Sugar: 29.5g

Day 27- Lunch: Low-FODMAP Tuna Salad Lettuce Wraps

Description: A light and refreshing lunch option featuring tuna salad wrapped in crisp lettuce leaves.

Preparation and Cooking Time: 10 minutes

Number of Servings: 4

Ingredients:
- 2 (5 oz) cans white tuna in water, drained and flaked
- 1/4 cup plain mayonnaise
- 1/4 cup celery, finely chopped
- 1/4 cup red bell pepper, finely diced
- 2 tbsp green onions (green tops only), chopped
- 1/3 pc lemon, juiced

- Salt and pepper, to taste
- 8 large lettuce leaves (Bibb, Boston, or iceberg)

Directions:

- In a medium bowl, combine the tuna, mayonnaise, celery, red bell pepper, green onion tops, and lemon juice. Season with salt and pepper to taste.
- Spoon the tuna salad evenly onto the center of each lettuce leaf.
- Fold the lettuce leaves around the tuna salad to form a wrap and enjoy.

Nutrition Information (per serving): Calories: 190, Protein: 17.1g, Fat: 12.2g, Carbohydrates: 2g, Fiber: 0.5g, Sugar: 0.9g

Day 27- Dinner: Low-FODMAP Eggplant Parmesan with Spaghetti Squash

Description: A comforting and delicious eggplant Parmesan served over a bed of roasted spaghetti squash.

Preparation and Cooking Time: 1 hour 10 minutes

Number of Servings: 4

Ingredients:

- 1 large spaghetti squash, halved and seeded
- 2 tbsp garlic-infused olive oil, divided
- Salt and pepper, to taste
- 1 medium eggplant, sliced into 1/4-inch rounds
- 1 cup gluten-free breadcrumbs
- 1/2 cup Parmesan cheese, grated
- 1 tsp dried basil
- 1 tsp dried oregano

- 1 large egg, beaten
- 2 cups low-FODMAP marinara sauce
- 1 1/2 cups mozzarella cheese, shredded

Directions:
- Preheat the oven to 400°F (200°C).
- Brush the cut sides of the spaghetti squash with 1 tablespoon of garlic-infused olive oil and season with salt and pepper. Place the squash halves cut-side down on a baking sheet and roast for 40-45 minutes, or until the squash is tender and can be easily scraped into strands with a fork.
- While the squash is roasting, prepare the eggplant Parmesan. In a shallow dish, combine the gluten-free breadcrumbs, Parmesan cheese, basil, and oregano.
- Dip each eggplant slice into the beaten egg, then coat with the breadcrumb mixture, pressing the breadcrumbs onto the eggplant to adhere.
- Heat the remaining 1 tablespoon of garlic-infused olive oil in a large skillet over medium heat. Cook the breaded eggplant slices for 3-4 minutes per side, or until golden brown and crisp.
- Spoon a thin layer of marinara sauce into the bottom of a baking dish. Arrange the cooked eggplant slices in a single layer over the sauce, then top with the remaining marinara sauce and shredded mozzarella cheese.
- Bake the eggplant Parmesan for 20-25 minutes, or until the cheese is melted and bubbly.
- Scrape the cooked spaghetti squash into strands and divide it among four plates. Top each serving with a portion of eggplant Parmesan and serve.

Note: In choosing marinara sauce, check the ingredient's nutrition label list. Watch out for onion or garlic since these ingredients have high FODMAP content.

Nutrition Information (per serving): Calories: 542, Protein: 27.5g, Fat: 25.7g, Carbohydrates: 56.9g, Fiber: 7.8g, Sugar: 8.9g

Day 28

Day 28- Breakfast: Low-FODMAP Green Smoothie

Description: A refreshing and nutritious green smoothie packed with fruits and vegetables.

Preparation and Cooking Time: 5 minutes

Number of Servings: 1

Ingredients:
- 1 cup spinach
- 1/2 cup diced pineapple
- 1/2 cup diced kiwi
- 1 small "just ripe" banana
- 1 cup unsweetened almond milk

Directions:
- In a blender, combine the spinach, pineapple, kiwi, banana, and almond milk. Blend until smooth and creamy.
- Pour the smoothie into a glass and enjoy.

Nutrition Information (per serving): Calories: 232, Protein: 4.4g, Fat: 4.5g, Carbohydrates: 50g, Fiber: 8.1g, Sugar: 28.6g

Day 28- Lunch: Low-FODMAP Greek Salad with Grilled Chicken

Description: A flavorful and satisfying Greek salad with juicy grilled chicken for added protein.

Preparation and Cooking Time: 20 minutes

Number of Servings: 4

Ingredients:

- 1 lb or 4 grilled chicken breasts, sliced
- 4 cups Romaine lettuce, chopped
- 1 cup cherry tomatoes, halved
- 1 cup cucumber, diced
- 1/2 cup Kalamata olives, pitted
- 1/2 cup feta cheese, crumbled
- 1/4 cup fresh parsley, chopped
- 1/4 cup garlic-infused olive oil
- 3 tbsp red wine vinegar
- Salt and pepper, to taste

Directions:

- In a large salad bowl, combine the Romaine lettuce, cherry tomatoes, cucumber, Kalamata olives, feta cheese, and fresh parsley.
- In a small bowl, whisk together the garlic-infused olive oil and red wine vinegar. Season with salt and pepper to taste.
- Drizzle the dressing over the salad and toss to combine.
- Top the salad with the sliced grilled chicken and serve immediately.

Nutrition Information (per serving): Calories: 393, Protein: 32.9g, Fat: 26.3g, Carbohydrates: 6.5g, Fiber: 1.7g, Sugar: 3g

Day 28- Dinner: Low-FODMAP Zucchini Noodle Stir-Fry with Chicken

Description: A light and delicious zucchini noodle stir-fry with tender chicken and a flavorful sauce.

Preparation and Cooking Time: 25 minutes

Number of Servings: 4

Ingredients:

- 2 medium zucchini, spiralized
- 1 tbsp garlic-infused olive oil
- 1 lb boneless, skinless chicken breasts, thinly sliced
- 1 cup carrots, julienned
- 1 cup red bell pepper, diced
- 1/4 cup low-sodium soy sauce (gluten-free)
- 2 tbsp rice vinegar
- 2 tbsp maple syrup
- 1 tbsp cornstarch
- Salt and pepper, to taste
- 2 tbsp green onions (green tops only), chopped, for garnish

Directions:

- Using a spiralizer, turn the zucchini into noodles. Set aside.
- In a large skillet or wok, heat the garlic-infused olive oil over medium-high heat. Add the chicken and cook for 4-5 minutes on each side, or until cooked through. Remove the chicken from the skillet and set aside.
- In the same skillet, add the carrots and red bell pepper, cooking for 3-4 minutes, or until the vegetables are tender-crisp.
- In a small bowl, whisk together the soy sauce, rice vinegar, maple syrup, and cornstarch. Pour the sauce into the skillet with the vegetables, stirring to coat. Cook for 1-2 minutes, or until the sauce has thickened slightly.

- Return the cooked chicken to the skillet and add the zucchini noodles. Toss to combine and heat through, then season with salt and pepper to taste.
- Serve the zucchini noodle stir-fry in bowls, garnished with chopped green onion tops.

Nutrition Information (per serving): Calories: 235, Protein: 29.2g, Fat: 5.3g, Carbohydrates: 18.5g, Fiber: 2.4g, Sugar: 11.8g

References

Chapter 1

- Chey WD, et al. Irritable bowel syndrome: a clinical review. JAMA. 2015 Mar 3;313(9):949-58.

- Lacy BE, et al. ACG Clinical Guideline: Management of Irritable Bowel Syndrome. Am J Gastroenterol. 2021 Jan 1;116(1):17-44.

- Liu H, et al. Prevalence and Influencing Factors of Irritable Bowel Syndrome in Medical Staff: A Meta-Analysis. Dig Dis Sci. 2022 Nov;67(11):5019-5028.

- Shin A, et al. The Prevalence, Humanistic Burden, and Health Care Impact of Irritable Bowel Syndrome Among United States Veterans. Clin Gastroenterol Hepatol. 2023 Apr;21(4):1061-1069.

- Oka P, et al. Global prevalence of irritable bowel syndrome according to Rome III or IV criteria: a systematic review and meta-analysis. Lancet Gastroenterol Hepatol. 2020 Oct;5(10):908-917.

Chapter 2

- Aaron LA, et al. Overlapping conditions among patients with chronic fatigue syndrome, fibromyalgia, and temporomandibular disorder. Arch Intern Med. 2000 Jan 24;160(2):221-7.

- Cámara-Lemarroy CR, et al. Gastrointestinal disorders associated with migraine: A comprehensive review. World J Gastroenterol. 2016 Sep 28;22(36):8149-60.

- Fond G, et al. Anxiety and depression comorbidities in irritable bowel syndrome (IBS): a systematic review and meta-analysis. Eur Arch Psychiatry Clin Neurosci. 2014 Dec;264(8):651-60.

- van Hemert S, et al. Migraine associated with gastrointestinal disorders: review of the literature and clinical implications. Front Neurol. 2014 Nov 21;5:241.

- Lee C, et al. Brain-Gut Axis Research Group of Korean Society of Neurogastroenterology and Motility. The Increased Level of Depression and Anxiety in Irritable Bowel Syndrome Patients Compared with Healthy Controls: Systematic Review and Meta-analysis. J Neurogastroenterol Motil. 2017 Jul 30;23(3):349-362.

- Sibelli A, et al. A systematic review with meta-analysis of the role of anxiety and depression in irritable bowel syndrome onset. Psychol Med. 2016 Nov;46(15):3065-3080.

- Hu Z, et al. The level and prevalence of depression and anxiety among patients with different subtypes of irritable bowel syndrome: a network meta-analysis. BMC Gastroenterol. 2021 Jan 7;21(1):23.

- Sperber AD, et al. Fibromyalgia in the irritable bowel syndrome: studies of prevalence and clinical implications. Am J Gastroenterol. 1999 Dec;94(12):3541-6.

Chapter 3

- Camilleri M, et al. Brain-gut axis: from basic understanding to treatment of IBS and related disorders. J Pediatr Gastroenterol Nutr. 2012 Apr;54(4):446-53.

- Saito YA, et al. Familial Aggregation of Irritable Bowel Syndrome: A Family Case-Control Study. Am J Gastroenterol. 2010;105(4):833-41.

- Ohman L, et al. Pathogenesis of IBS: role of inflammation, immunity and neuroimmune interactions. Nat Rev Gastroenterol Hepatol. 2010 Mar;7(3):163-73.

- Park SH, et al. Adverse childhood experiences are associated with irritable bowel syndrome and gastrointestinal symptom severity. Neurogastroenterology & Motility. 2016 Aug;28(8):1252-60.

- Bonfiglio F, et al. Female-Specific Association Between Variants on Chromosome 9 and Self-Reported Diagnosis of Irritable Bowel Syndrome. Gastroenterology. 2018;155(1):168-179.

- Makker J, et al. Genetic epidemiology of irritable bowel syndrome. World journal of gastroenterology vol. 21,40 (2015): 11353-61.

- van Thiel I, et al. Fungal feelings in the irritable bowel syndrome: the intestinal mycobiome and abdominal pain. Gut Microbes. 2023 Jan-Dec;15(1):2168992.

- Dinan TG, et al. The Microbiome-Gut-Brain Axis in Health and Disease. Gastroenterol Clin North Am. 2017 Mar;46(1):77-89.

- Drossman DA. Functional Gastrointestinal Disorders: History, Pathophysiology, Clinical Features and Rome IV. Gastroenterology. 2016 Feb 19:S0016-5085(16)00223-7.

- Okafor PN, et al. Environmental Pollutants Are Associated with Irritable Bowel Syndrome in a Commercially Insured Cohort of California Residents. Clin Gastroenterol Hepatol. 2022 Oct 3:S1542-3565(22)00923-5.

- Spiller RC. Postinfectious irritable bowel syndrome. Gastroenterology. 2003 Apr;124(4):1662-71.

- Jeffery IB, et al. An irritable bowel syndrome subtype defined by species-specific alterations in faecal microbiota. Gut. 2012 Jul;61(7):997-1006.

- Goodoory VC, et al. Systematic Review and Meta-analysis: Efficacy of Mesalamine in Irritable Bowel Syndrome. Clin Gastroenterol Hepatol. 2023 Feb 27:S1542-3565(23)00156-8.

- Mayer EA. Gut feelings: the emerging biology of gut-brain communication. Nat Rev Neurosci. 2011 Jul 6;12(8):453-66.

- Jalanka J, et al. Postinfective bowel dysfunction following *Campylobacter enteritis* is characterised by reduced microbiota diversity and impaired microbiota recovery. Gut. 2023 Mar;72(3):451-459.

- Marasco G, et al. GI-COVID19 study group. Post COVID-19 irritable bowel syndrome. Gut. 2022 Dec 9:gutjnl-2022-328483.
- Camilleri M. Leaky gut: mechanisms, measurement and clinical implications in humans. Gut. 2019 Aug;68(8):1516-1526.
- Zhou Q, et al. Randomised placebo-controlled trial of dietary glutamine supplements for postinfectious irritable bowel syndrome. Gut. 2019 Jun;68(6):996-1002.

Chapter 4
- Veale D, et al. Primary fibromyalgia and the irritable bowel syndrome: different expressions of a common pathogenetic process. Br J Rheumatol. 1991 Jun;30(3):220-2.

Chapter 5
- Kinsinger SW. Practical Approaches to Working with a Gastrointestinal Psychologist. Gastroenterol Clin North Am. 2022 Dec;51(4):711-721.
- McDonald E, et al. A Randomized Trial of a Group-Based Integrative Medicine Approach Compared to Waitlist Control on Irritable Bowel Syndrome Symptoms in Adults. Explore (NY). 2018 Nov;14(6):406-413.
- Chey WD, et al. Behavioral and Diet Therapies in Integrated Care for Patients With Irritable Bowel Syndrome. Gastroenterology. 2021 Jan;160(1):47-62.

Chapter 6
- Chey WD, et al. AGA Clinical Practice Update on the Role of Diet in Irritable Bowel Syndrome: Expert Review. Gastroenterology. 2022 May;162(6):1737-1745.
- Dionne J, et al. A Systematic Review and Meta-Analysis Evaluating the Efficacy of a Gluten-Free Diet and a Low FODMAPs Diet in Treating Symptoms of Irritable Bowel Syndrome. Am J Gastroenterol. 2018 Sep;113(9):1290-1300.

- Black CJ, et al. Efficacy of a low FODMAP diet in irritable bowel syndrome: systematic review and network meta-analysis. Gut. 2022 Jun;71(6):1117-1126.

- Bijkerk CJ, et al. Soluble or insoluble fibre in irritable bowel syndrome in primary care? Randomised placebo controlled trial. BMJ. 2009 Aug 27;339:b3154.

- Ford AC, et al. Effect of fibre, antispasmodics, and peppermint oil in the treatment of irritable bowel syndrome: systematic review and meta-analysis. BMJ. 2008 Nov 13;337

- Vazquez-Roque, Maria I et al. "A controlled trial of gluten-free diet in patients with irritable bowel syndrome-diarrhea: effects on bowel frequency and intestinal function." *Gastroenterology* vol. 144,5 2013: 903-911.

- Shahbazkhani B, et al. Non-Celiac Gluten Sensitivity Has Narrowed the Spectrum of Irritable Bowel Syndrome: A Double-Blind Randomized Placebo-Controlled Trial. Nutrients. 2015 Jun 5;7(6):4542-54.

- Moayyedi P, et al. The effect of fiber supplementation on irritable bowel syndrome: a systematic review and meta-analysis. Am J Gastroenterol. 2014 Sep;109(9):1367-74.

- Böhn L, et al. Diet low in FODMAPs reduces symptoms of irritable bowel syndrome as well as traditional dietary advice: a randomized controlled trial. Gastroenterology. 2015 Nov;149(6):1399-1407.

- Staudacher HM, et al. Fermentable carbohydrate restriction reduces luminal bifidobacteria and gastrointestinal symptoms in patients with irritable bowel syndrome. J Nutr. 2012;142(8):1510-1518.

- Ohlsson B. Theories behind the effect of starch and sucrose-reduced diets on gastrointestinal symptoms in irritable bowel syndrome (Review). Mol Med Rep. 2021 Oct;24(4):732.

- Nilholm, Clara et al. "A Dietary Intervention with Reduction of Starch and Sucrose Leads to Reduced Gastrointestinal and

Extra-Intestinal Symptoms in IBS Patients." *Nutrients* vol. 11,7
1662. 20 Jul. 2019

- Lovell RM, et al. Global prevalence of and risk factors for irritable bowel syndrome: a meta-analysis. Clin Gastroenterol Hepatol. 2012;10(7):712-721.e4.

- Drossman DA, et al. Severity in irritable bowel syndrome: a Rome Foundation Working Team report. Am J Gastroenterol. 2011;106(10):1749-1759; quiz 1760.

Chapter 7

- Lackner, J. M., et al. Improvement in gastrointestinal symptoms after cognitive behavior therapy for refractory irritable bowel syndrome. Gastroenterology, 2011. 141(1), 36-42.

- Everitt, H. A., et al. Assessing telephone-delivered cognitive-behavioural therapy (CBT) and web-delivered CBT versus treatment as usual in irritable bowel syndrome (ACTIB): A multicentre randomised trial. Gut, 2019. 68(9), 1613-1623.

- Black CJ, et al. Efficacy of psychological therapies for irritable bowel syndrome: systematic review and network meta-analysis. Gut. 2020 Aug;69(8):1441-1451.

- Everitt H, et al. Therapist telephone-delivered CBT and web-based CBT compared with treatment as usual in refractory irritable bowel syndrome: the ACTIB three-arm RCT. Health Technol Assess. 2019 Apr;23(17):1-154.

- Whorwell, et al. Controlled trial of hypnotherapy in the treatment of severe refractory irritable-bowel syndrome. Lancet, 1984. 2(8414), 1232-1234.

- Gonsalkorale, et al. Hypnotherapy in irritable bowel syndrome: a large-scale audit of a clinical service with examination of factors influencing responsiveness. The American Journal of Gastroenterology, 2002. 97(4), 954-961.

- Peters SL,et al. Smartphone app-delivered gut-directed hypnotherapy improves symptoms of self-reported irritable bowel syndrome: A retrospective evaluation. Neurogastroenterol Motil. 2023 Apr;35(4):e14533.

- Gaylord, S. A., et al. Mindfulness training reduces the severity of irritable bowel syndrome in women: results of a randomized controlled trial. The American Journal of Gastroenterology, 2011. 106(9), 1678-1688.

- Zernicke, K. A., et al. Mindfulness-based stress reduction for the treatment of irritable bowel syndrome symptoms: a randomized wait-list controlled trial. International Journal of Behavioral Medicine, 2013. 20(3), 385-396.

- Gerson J, et al. Patients' experiences with virtual group gut-directed hypnotherapy: A qualitative study. Front Med (Lausanne). 2023 Feb 22;10:1066452.

- Schumann, D., et al. Effect of Yoga in the Therapy of Irritable Bowel Syndrome: A Systematic Review. Clinical Gastroenterology and Hepatology, 2016. 14(12), 1720-1731.

- D'Silva A, et al. Yoga as a Therapy for Irritable Bowel Syndrome. Dig Dis Sci. 2020 Sep;65(9):2503-2514.

- Johannesson, E., et al. Physical activity improves symptoms in irritable bowel syndrome: a randomized controlled trial. The American Journal of Gastroenterology, 2011. 106(5), 915-922.

- Gaylord SA, et al. Mindfulness training reduces the severity of irritable bowel syndrome in women: results of a randomized controlled trial. Am J Gastroenterol. 2011 Sep;106(9):1678-88.

- Kearney DJ, et al. Effects of participation in a mindfulness program for veterans with posttraumatic stress disorder: a randomized controlled pilot study. J Clin Psychol. 2013 Jan;69(1):14-27.

- Cammarota G, et al. Randomised clinical trial: faecal microbiota transplantation by colonoscopy vs. vancomycin for the treatment of recurrent Clostridium difficile infection. Aliment Pharmacol Ther. 2015 May;41(9):835-43.

Chapter 8

- Saps M, et al. Multicenter, randomized, placebo-controlled trial of amitriptyline in children with functional gastrointestinal disorders. Gastroenterology. 2009 Oct;137(4):1261-9.

- Ford, A. C., et al. Efficacy of prebiotics, probiotics, and synbiotics in irritable bowel syndrome and chronic idiopathic constipation: systematic review and meta-analysis. The American journal of gastroenterology, 2014. 109(10), 1547.

- Cash, B., et al. A novel delivery system of peppermint oil is an effective therapy for irritable bowel syndrome symptoms. Digestive diseases and sciences, 2016. 61(2), 560-571.

- Rao, Satish S C, et al. Efficacy and Safety of Over-the-Counter Therapies for Chronic Constipation: An Updated Systematic Review. *The American journal of gastroenterology* vol. 116,6 (2021): 1156-1181.

- Ruepert L, et al. Bulking agents, antispasmodics and antidepressants for the treatment of irritable bowel syndrome. Cochrane Database Syst Rev. 2011 Aug 10;2011(8).

- Ingrosso MR, et al. Systematic review and meta-analysis: efficacy of peppermint oil in irritable bowel syndrome. Aliment Pharmacol Ther. 2022 Sep;56(6):932-941.

- Madisch A, et al. Treatment of irritable bowel syndrome with herbal preparations: results of a double-blind, randomized, placebo-controlled, multi-centre trial. Aliment Pharmacol Ther. 2004 Feb 1;19(3):271-9.

- Xie C, et al. Efficacy and Safety of Antidepressants for the Treatment of Irritable Bowel Syndrome: A Meta-Analysis. PLoS One. 2015 Aug 7;10(8).

- Ruepert, L., et al. Bulking agents, antispasmodics and antidepressants for the treatment of irritable bowel syndrome. Cochrane Database Syst Rev. 2011 Aug 10;2011(8).

- Lembo, A. J., et al. (2012). Linaclotide for irritable bowel syndrome with constipation: a 26-week, randomized, double-blind, placebo-controlled trial to evaluate efficacy and safety. The American Journal of Gastroenterology, 107(11), 1702-1712.

- Lembo, A. J., et al. Eluxadoline for Irritable Bowel Syndrome with Diarrhea. New England Journal of Medicine, 2016. 374(3), 242-253.

- Pimentel, M., et al. Rifaximin therapy for patients with irritable bowel syndrome without constipation. New England Journal of Medicine, 2011. 364(1), 22-32.

- Camilleri, M., et al. Efficacy and safety of alosetron in women with irritable bowel syndrome: a randomised, placebo-controlled trial. Lancet, 2000. 355(9209), 1035-1040.

Chapter 9

- Khanna R, et al. Peppermint oil for the treatment of irritable bowel syndrome: a systematic review and meta-analysis. J Clin Gastroenterol. 2014 Jul;48(6):505-12.

- Ford AC, et al. Systematic review with meta-analysis: the efficacy of prebiotics, probiotics, synbiotics and antibiotics in irritable bowel syndrome. Aliment Pharmacol Ther. 2018 Nov;48(10):1044-1060.

- Ford AC, et al. Efficacy of prebiotics, probiotics, and synbiotics in irritable bowel syndrome and chronic idiopathic constipation: systematic review and meta-analysis. Am J Gastroenterol. 2014 Oct;109(10):1547-61.

- Niu HL, et al. The efficacy and safety of probiotics in patients with irritable bowel syndrome: Evidence based on 35 randomized controlled trials. Int J Surg. 2020 Mar;75:116-127.

- Didari T, et al. Effectiveness of probiotics in irritable bowel syndrome: Updated systematic review with meta-analysis. World J Gastroenterol. 2015 Mar 14;21(10):3072-84.

- Wang XY, et al. Acupuncture for functional gastrointestinal disorders: A systematic review and meta-analysis. J Gastroenterol Hepatol. 2021 Nov;36(11):3015-3026.

- Wang L, et al. Acupuncture for emotional symptoms in patients with functional gastrointestinal disorders: A systematic review and meta-analysis. PLoS One. 2022 Jan 27;17(1).

- Zheng, Hui et al. "Chinese Herbal Medicine for Irritable Bowel Syndrome: A Meta-Analysis and Trial Sequential Analysis of Randomized Controlled Trials." *Frontiers in pharmacology* vol. 12 694741. 27 Jul. 2021

- Faghih Dinevari M, et al. The effect of melatonin on irritable bowel syndrome patients with and without sleep disorders: a randomized double-blinded placebo-controlled trial study. BMC Gastroenterol. 2023 Apr 25;23(1):135.

- Naik TD, Tubaki BR, Patankar DS. Efficacy of whole system ayurveda protocol in irritable bowel syndrome - A Randomized controlled clinical trial. J Ayurveda Integr Med. 2023 Jan-Feb;14(1):100592.

- Peckham EJ, et al. Homeopathy for treatment of irritable bowel syndrome. Cochrane Database Syst Rev. 2013 Nov 13;(11):CD009710.

- Dai YQ, et al. Moxibustion for diarrhea-predominant irritable bowel syndrome: A systematic review and meta-analysis of randomized controlled trials. Complement Ther Clin Pract. 2022 Feb;46:101532.

Chapter 10

- Cangemi DJ, et al. A Practical Approach to the Diagnosis and Treatment of Abdominal Bloating and Distension. Gastroenterol Hepatol (N Y). 2022 Feb;18(2):75-84.

Chapter 11

- Camacho S, et al. Sexual dysfunction worsens both the general and specific quality of life of women with irritable bowel syndrome. A cross-sectional study. BMC Womens Health. 2023 Mar 27;23(1):134.

- Cockrum R, Tu F. Hysterectomy for Chronic Pelvic Pain. Obstet Gynecol Clin North Am. 2022 Jun;49(2):257-271.

- Latthe P, et al. WHO systematic review of prevalence of chronic pelvic pain: a neglected reproductive health morbidity. BMC Public Health. 2006 Jul 6;6:177.

- Matheis A, et al. Irritable bowel syndrome and chronic pelvic pain: a singular or two different clinical syndrome? World J Gastroenterol. 2007 Jul 7;13(25):3446-55.

- Mathias SD, et al. Chronic pelvic pain: prevalence, health-related quality of life, and economic correlates. Obstet Gynecol. 1996 Mar;87(3):321-7.

- Johnson CM, et al. Fibromyalgia and Irritable Bowel Syndrome in Female Pelvic Pain. Semin Reprod Med. 2018 Mar;36(2):136-142.

Chapter 16

- Linsalata M, et al. Somatization is associated with altered serum levels of vitamin D, serotonin, and brain-derived neurotrophic factor in patients with predominant diarrhea irritable bowel syndrome. Neurogastroenterol Motil. 2023 Mar;35(3):e14512.

- Körner E, et al. Fecal microbiota transplantation in patients with irritable bowel syndrome: an overview of current studies. J Appl Microbiol. 2023 Mar 7

- Spiegel BMR, et al. Qualitative Validation of a Novel VR Program for Irritable Bowel Syndrome: A VR1 Study. Am J Gastroenterol. 2022 Mar 1;117(3):495-500.

- Deng X, et al. Intestinal crosstalk between bile acids and microbiota in irritable bowel syndrome. J Gastroenterol Hepatol. 2023. doi: 10.1111/jgh.16159.

- Min YW, et al. Bile Acid and Gut Microbiota in Irritable Bowel Syndrome. J Neurogastroenterol Motil. 2022 Oct 30;28(4):549-561.

- Bonfiglio F., et al. Female-specific association between variants on chromosome 9 and self-reported diagnosis of irritable bowel syndrome. Gastroenterology. 2018 Jul;155(1):168-179.

- Tkach S, et al. Fecal microbiota transplantation in patients with post-infectious irritable bowel syndrome: A randomized, clinical trial. Front Med (Lausanne). 2022 Oct 20;9:994911.

- Karakan T, et al. Artificial intelligence-based personalized diet: A pilot clinical study for irritable bowel syndrome. Gut Microbes. 2022 Jan-Dec;14(1):2138672.

- Dao VH, et al. Psychobiotics for Patients with Chronic Gastrointestinal Disorders Having Anxiety or Depression Symptoms. J Multidiscip Healthc. 2021 Jun 10;14:1395-1402.

- Algladi T, et al. Modulation of human visceral sensitivity by noninvasive magnetoelectrical neural stimulation in health and irritable bowel syndrome. Pain. 2015 Jul;156(7):1348-1356.

- Gentile, M et al. Innovative approaches to service integration addressing the unmet needs of irritable bowel syndrome patients and new approaches for the needs of IBS patients. *Frontiers in medicine* vol. 9 998838. 16 Nov. 2022.

- Rao SSC, et al. Randomized Placebo-Controlled Phase 3 Trial of Vibrating Capsule for Chronic Constipation. Gastroenterology. 2023 Feb 21:S0016-5085(23)00149-X.

- Zhu JH, et al. Efficacy and safety of vibrating capsule for functional constipation (VICONS): A randomised, double-blind, placebo-controlled, multicenter trial. EClinicalMedicine. 2022 Apr 25;47:101407.

About the Author

Sripathi Kethu, M.D. is a seasoned physician with over 30 years of experience in the medical field specializing in gastroenterology. He completed his clinical gastroenterology fellowship at Brown University. He received advanced training in endoscopy at the Institute Paoli-Calmettes in Marseille, France. Following his training, he served as an Assistant Professor at Brown University. He is a Diplomate of the American Board of Internal Medicine in Internal Medicine and Gastroenterology. He is a fellow of American College of Gastroenterology and American Society of Gastrointestinal Endoscopy.

Dr. Kethu is a highly respected member of the medical community, with extensive experience publishing research articles in clinical journals, authoring textbook chapters, and writing informative blog posts on a range of healthcare topics, including digestive health. He is currently in private gastroenterology practice in Dallas, where he continues to help patients manage their gastrointestinal conditions. He has been voted by his peers as D-magazine's one of the best Gastroenterologists in Dallas 10 years in a row.

Outside of his professional life, Dr. Kethu is an accomplished athlete and an avid outdoor enthusiast. He has tackled many challenges, including trekking to Mount Everest Base Camp, completing the Hotter'N Hell 100-mile bike ride, and taking part in the 150-mile MS 150 bike rides to raise funds for multiple sclerosis research and support services. He is also a passionate runner who has completed marathons in all 50 states of the USA and on all seven continents, including

Antarctica. He even earned the highly coveted Six Star Abbott Majors Medal for finishing all six Abbott World Marathon Majors.

In his personal life, Dr. Kethu cherishes his time with his physician wife and their two wonderful daughters, enjoying the love and support they share as a family.

With his vast experience, dedication to health, and passion for adventure, Dr. Kethu provides a unique perspective and invaluable insights into IBS and overall wellness.

Printed in Great Britain
by Amazon